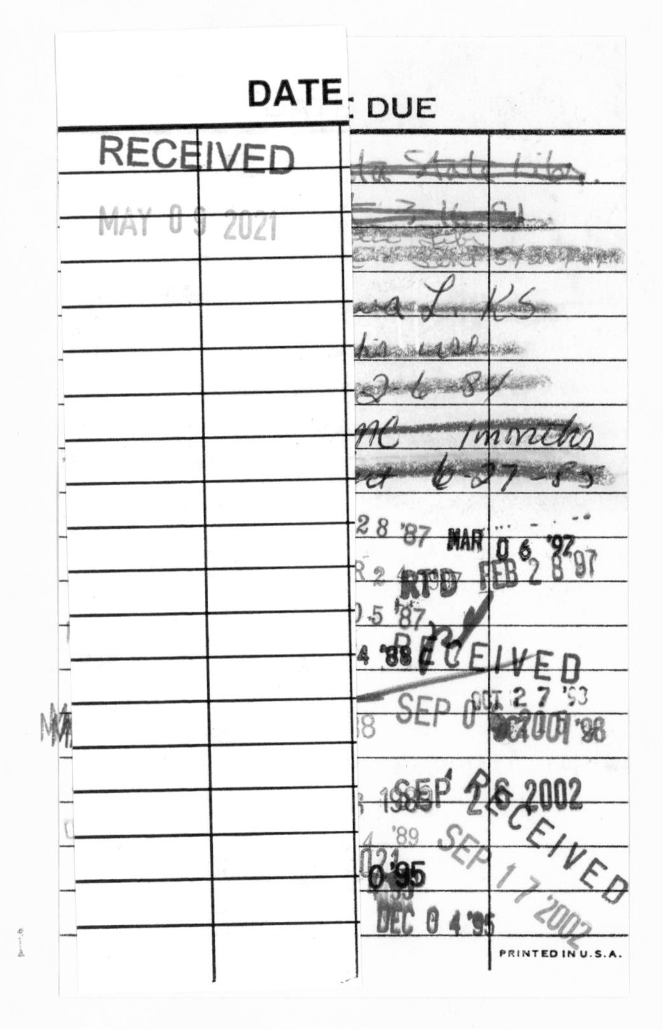
DATE DUE
RECEIVED
MAY 0 9 2021
PRINTED IN U.S.A.

Too Old To Cry, Too Young To Die

TOO OLD TO CRY, TOO YOUNG TO DIE

35 Teenagers Talk About Cancer

Compiled by

EDITH PENDLETON

Thomas Nelson Publishers
Nashville

Library of Congress Cataloging in Publication Data:

Pendleton, Edith.
Too old to cry, too young to die.

1. Cancer—Patients—Biography.
2. Tumors in teenagers—Biography. I. Title.
RC263.P34 362.1'96994 80–18463
ISBN 0–8407–4086–7

Contents

Introduction

Jill Chapman called it a quickie course in growing up. Having cancer, at any age, is certainly that. It can play havoc with priorities, printing its name across every thought.

For people in their teens and early twenties, it can impose special complications: How do you explain it to friends? How do you *keep from* explaining it to friends, dates, teachers, curious neighbors, brothers and sisters? And where in all life's dictionary are the words that explain "Why me?"

They're not printed here. Instead, this book records the experiences of thirty-five teens and young adults who have had cancer. Some offer advice; some simply explain what has happened to them.

The project was inspired by a panel of teenagers who spoke at the national conference of Candlelighters, a parents' support group, in the spring of 1978. Their remarks provided the first actual transcripts for the book.

A few months later, I attended an unusual two-week summer camp for kids with cancer held near Shands Teaching Hospital in Gainesville, Florida. There, as fast as the kids talked, I tape-recorded them, then sat on a bunk and transcribed what they'd said. As fast as the pages rolled out, they edited them and added topics for later discussions. There seemed little doubt in anybody's mind that we *really were* writing a book.

When camp closed, I drove cross-country, covering Georgia, Alabama, Missouri, and fringes of North Carolina, interviewing kids with cancer. Many times I sacked out on living-room floors or in the back seat of my car. Friends sometimes put me up; oftentimes I stayed in hospital rooms with kids who talked when the spirit moved them. So, at long last, here's what they had to say.

YOU HAVE WHAT?
IT ALL ADDS UP
TO CANCER

Leukemia

Leukemia is the most common form of cancer found in children. It strikes suddenly, infiltrating the bone marrow with abnormal and immature white blood cells. For this reason, it is sometimes called cancer of the blood.

As recently as five years ago, leukemia was considered incurable. Today, particularly in children, it has one of the highest cure rates known for cancer.

There are several types of leukemia, but all involve the production of abnormal leukocytes, white blood cells formed in the spongy interior of the bone called the marrow. Without these vital blood components, the body becomes highly vulnerable to infection and hemorrhage (bleeding). Damaged most are the platelets, the blood components necessary for clotting.

The two most common forms of leukemia are acute lymphocytic leukemia (A.L.L.) and chronic leukemia. A.L.L. strikes children most; chronic leukemia (less than half of all cases) occurs generally in adults.

Treatment involves a sequence of four or more drugs, all of which kill leukemic cells, but which have different damaging effects on normal cells. The spread of cancer cells to the central nervous system is stopped by methotrexate injected into the spinal column and by radiation to the head. After the first large doses, smaller amounts of the drug are continued for several years to wipe out any new but undetected leukemic cells.

Patients also receive injections of vincristine to stop cell division; of prednisone to suppress white blood cell formation; and later, of l-asparaginase, an enzyme produced by the common intestinal bacterium E. coli.

Maintenance therapy usually lasts five years. Spinal taps and strong doses of vincristine from time to time serve to keep the disease at bay. After five years, if there are no signs of leukemia in the blood, therapy is stopped.

Hodgkin's Disease

"People react in strange ways when they hear you have Hodgkin's," says Millie Thomas, thirteen.

"If they've never heard of it, they don't know how to approach you. They get it confused with something else, or refer to some distant friend of a cousin who had something like that."

Hodgkin's disease is a form of cancer that originates in the lymphatic system—the tiny lymph glands in the neck, the armpits, and the groin. These bean-sized glands produce the white blood cells that fight infection. As the Hodgkin's progresses, the body becomes less able to fight germs. The first symptoms aren't much different from those associated with a sore throat or the flu.

But when the lymph glands remain swollen for three weeks or more, the case may seem suspicious. By taking X rays a physician can determine the stage of the disease and how far it has spread.

Then, by taking a microscopic slice of tissue from the diseased area, known as a biopsy, the Hodgkin's can be diagnosed. From the biopsy, the pathologist (a doctor trained to spot microscopic changes in tissues) then classifies the disease by its "stage."

If the disease is confined to one lymph area, it is classed as Stage 1. If it has spread to adjacent lymph regions but is confined to one half of the body, it is called Stage 2. Stages 3 and 4 identify more serious cases. Each of the various stages is further subdivided into groups A and B according to the symptoms the patient experiences.

Sometimes doctors inject a radiopaque dye (one which shows up on X rays) into the lymph system of the patient. This procedure is called a lymph-angiography. When the patient is then X-rayed, the stage of the disease can be determined by studying the negatives of the lymph system.

Intense X ray treatments to each lymph node region involved has been the most common and effective treatment for early Hodgkin's disease.

According to the Office of Cancer Communications in Bethesda, Maryland, more extensive preventive radiotherapy (treatment with X rays) has produced promising results. With this technique, high doses of radiotherapy are delivered to all lymph nodes in the torso, rather than only to those nodes known to be diseased. This tactic could slow down a recurrence of the disease in other nodes beyond the original site of the disease.

A four-drug combination is generally used on more advanced Hodgkin's disease patients. These include nitrogen mustard and related alkylating agents; vinblastine and vincristine, both made from extracts of the periwinkle plant; methyl hydrazine derivative or procarbazine; and methotrexate. Prednisone has also been used with success.

Wilms's Tumor

Wilms's Tumor most often occurs in preschoolers but occasionally crops up in older children. The tumor begins in the kidney, where it grows so rapidly it may become quite large before it is detected.

If it is discovered soon enough, it can be treated with a combination of surgery, radiation, and chemotherapy. It is the most frequently cured form of childhood cancer.

Unfortunately, the tumor can break apart and travel through the blood stream, where it most often metastasizes (regroups) in the lungs.

Vincristine, Adriamycin, and postoperative radiation are the usual forms of treatment. If the tumor does not recur within two years, the patient is considered tentatively cured.

Osteogenic Sarcoma

This form of bone cancer, though rare, occurs most often in youth ten to twenty years old. It usually arises in the ends of long bones—the wrists, knees, and ankles—during the peak of the adolescent growth spurt.

It is one of the fastest moving cancers known. It begins in the bone, cartilage, and fibrous tissues, and in the past has required prompt amputation of the affected limb.

While surgery remains the most common treatment, some progress has been made in the implanting of stainless steel rods to replace diseased bone. The patient must be full-grown for the implantation to fit, and since it must be custom made, some degree of risk is involved for the patient who postpones surgery. Preoperative chemotherapy can begin destroying the primary tumor at once.

Other Types of Cancer

Neuroblastoma: This cancer affects the central nervous system. It is the second most common type of childhood cancer, next to leukemia. It arises in certain nerve fibers of the body, most commonly in the abdomen. It can be detected by a simple urine test; one of the first symptoms is a swelling of the abdomen. It strikes very young children and infants primarily. If detected early and treated, eighty percent of children are alive and well five years later. Unfortunately, more than half are undiagnosed until after the cancer spreads beyond the original site.

Brain Cancers: In younger children these cancers are difficult to detect, but with teens the symptoms are generally blurred or double vision, dizziness, difficulty in walking, and unexplained nausea and vomiting. Some brain cancers can be cured if treatment begins early.

Rhabdomyosarcoma: This cancer of the muscle tissue occurs almost anywhere in the body and for that reason is almost impossible to recognize from symptoms. It often spreads rapidly, metastasizing to lungs, bone, and other organs. As with other cancers occurring in the soft tissue, the size of the tumor plays a major part in determining the prognosis.

Retinoblastoma: This eye cancer usually occurs in children under four years old. The first symptom may be a widening of the pupil of the eye. Later a pearly glint, commonly called a cat's eye reflex, may show up. Surgery or radiation, sometimes in combination with drugs, can cure eighty-five percent of youngsters with this cancer. The vision in the affected eye can often be saved. This cancer runs in families, so that if one child in a family has developed it, others may also.

TALK ABOUT CANCER: NINE CASE HISTORIES

Jill Chapman

What do you tell a fourteen-year-old with Hodgkin's disease? That she's got a dislocated cold? A disease of the lymph nodes? A cluster of deformed cells? Jill Chapman heard everything but the raw fact: She had cancer.

It took four months before Jill realized what she had. Yet she remembers the misunderstanding as a coping mechanism that postponed the truth just long enough for her to regain her physical strength.

Now a college sophomore, she remembers her teens as a testing ground for self-esteem. "I used to tell people indiscriminately that I had cancer," she says. "I was trying so hard to make something of myself, to be somebody. By telling them how sick I'd been I felt I was saying, 'I know more about some things at fourteen than you may ever know.' "

Jill plans to become a counselor for children with catastrophic illnesses.

I was diagnosed with Hodgkin's disease when I was in the ninth grade. I was fourteen and president of the student council, which was a big deal.

But I was resentful, too, and in the middle of deciding about myself. I wished myself to be real sick so that I'd get a lot of attention and sympathy. Unfortunately, it was a self-fulfilling prophecy. I began to feel sick, and in about two months I had a lump in my neck. So they put me into the hospital. By that time, I was too tired to care.

They did a biopsy on the lymph nodes and told me I had Hodgkin's disease. I said, "Okay, what's that?" So they explained my lymph nodes to me and what they did and said I had a malignant tumor in my neck, but they never said the word "cancer." They told me all of it, but I never caught on that it was really cancer.

I think my parents had a lot of faith that I would figure it out sooner or later. But I had radiation treatments and went back to school in the fall still not knowing.

But a lot of people at school *did* know, and that was hard to deal with. Earlier, my dad had told one of my friends that he didn't know if I'd be back at school, period. Not just this year. Not ever. So when I went back my friends were all thinking I would die in two weeks, and I was saying, "What gave you that idea?"

I wasn't feeling very secure about what I knew. So I looked it up in the encyclopedia. The first thing I saw was, "*Hodgkin's disease:* a cancerous disease of the blah blah blah. . . ." I read it again. The whole thing. I was very calm about it. I thought, "Naw, couldn't be." I spent a lot of nights alone in my room figuring it out, saying, "Yes, you've got cancer. Yes you DO." And it was a long time even after that—at least six months—before I heard a doctor or my mother or anyone even say that word.

Looking back on it, I think that I was blessed with my ignorance. It got me through getting well. I always saw an end to being sick. But I really was a little taken aback to know it took me three months after they told me to realize what it really was.

The following summer I got sick again. They started giving me chemotherapy and cobalt at the same time. I have very weak veins, and sometimes they would fibrose—become hard and black and blue. It was so painful that it became as much an emotional struggle as it was a physical one to go in the clinic. At that time they only had hard aluminum folding chairs set up in a long hall, and it was very uncomfortable to have to sit there and wait. I would get so upset I'd actually feel sick.

Then one day a friend said, "Maybe you ought to think about why you're getting sick." I knew what she was saying. That I was getting sick in my mind. I went to work on it. It took discipline. But by the end of the treatments I was able to eat dinner and be relatively healthy all weekend after getting the medicine on Friday. I learned what I can do when I have to. I called it a "quickie course in growing up."

While I was on chemotherapy, I know I looked bad many of the times I went to school. I felt so bad I didn't notice it. Somehow it just didn't bother me.

The pills kept me constantly nauseous, so I didn't eat. And I couldn't wear skirts and dresses because I couldn't wear heels. I lost all the reflexes in my ankles, and I couldn't stand on my heels. My ankles were limp. I couldn't go up and down stairs unless I lifted my foot with my leg.

I wore these ugly green tennis shoes, guy's tennis shoes. They became my trademark. I'd come up the steps flop, flop, flop.

I remember I'd put a skirt on and look in the mirror, and the skirt would be longer in the back than in the front. I'd take the skirt off and lay it on the bed and match up the waist band so I knew that it was even. It wasn't longer in the back. And I'd put the stupid skirt on, and it'd still look long in the back. I'd lost so much weight there was nothing back there to hold the skirt up.

I was having problems with my leg, and I remember that my thigh looked so bad it bothered me. The muscle, instead of coming out, went in. I had a comparison—I could see how thin that thigh was compared to the other one. But that was just one part of me. When all of me got thin, I just ignored it.

But I became super-sensitive in another way: I suddenly realized things I had taken for granted, like being put down by somebody who didn't have to put me down. It became more important to me than it had been before. I acted upon it.

One day during lab class I noticed a kid with his feet up on a chair telling his friends, "Yeah, I took a pill to get up this morning, and I took a pill before lunch so I'd feel better; but then I had to take another pill so I could get back down so I could do my homework. But then I smoked grass last night, and then I had to take a pill so I could get up this morning."

That made me so mad I turned around and said, "You think that's really funny, don't you? Taking pills like that, ruining your life. Well, how would you like to have some nitrogen mustard. Oh, that's a real blast. You'd love that."

I was so embarrassed and so mad, I walked away. My knees were shaking. And that kid got up and walked over to me and said, "I didn't know. What's wrong?" And we talked. And he's still probably a good for nothing nobody, and I'm still a little whacky in *his* mind because I'd do that—but I'm glad I did.

But I have to bite my tongue a lot. It's like saving your fire. You can't get all worked up, especially when you think, "They aren't going to respond to what I have to say."

I used to tell people indiscriminately that I had cancer. It was such a big part of my life. I told people all the time. But many times as soon as I said the word "cancer" people assumed I was going to die, and they were overwhelmed. They didn't know what to do with that. So they just tuned me out, turned me off, talked about something else.

That made me mad, and I'd try to tell them that cancer isn't something you can ignore. It's a big problem that a lot of people have to face, that *they* might have to face some day.

I was having trouble communicating with my parents, too. Our big battle was over my freedom. When I first got sick they were real protective, and that was okay as long as I was sick. But when I didn't feel sick, I didn't see why I should have to act sick. They were telling me, "No, you should stay home and take good care of yourself," or "You're doing too much." One time I wanted to go to a Christmas party, and I had a fever. When you're sick you can't give up your social life. I know you have to restrict it. That's the hard part because parents can't know what's a restriction and what's going to really hurt a kid's social life. It's very important, and they can really mess things up for you. You have to maintain a normal life as far as possible. I was trying to be super-normal, and my parents were trying to make me pseudo-normal, less than normal. We needed a middle ground. I'd win a battle, but never a war. We compromised.

I always think the kids set the mood. At least *I* did. If I had said to my parents, "What should I do?" instead of taking the initiative myself and saying, "I'm going to do such and such," then they would have made the decisions and been protective parents all my life. I think if anything, I felt guilty for getting sick, and that's why I was so determined.

Just before I graduated from high school, my minister asked if I would like to go to Rhode Island for the summer, by myself, and do church work there the whole summer. He asked me and I said, "Yeah!" I don't know what possessed me to say that. I surprised myself, and when I talked to Mom she said, "You mean you told the preacher you could go and you hadn't even told us yet?" So it happens. It works out. That's the only way to learn—to ask questions, to guess, to try.

My parents put tremendous faith in me. They didn't deliver a death sentence to me. They did at first, but they came through for me. But they would never talk about the future. I didn't think about it, either. I wouldn't let myself think past the first semester of college. I didn't want to have a bunch of plans and then find out the future wasn't going to be there.

I expected so much from college. But I've found that, even at college, the kids are so dumb. They have to drink, because you can't have fun if you can't drink. I don't smoke, and I don't drink. I found out that can be hard when your date is sitting there trying to ignore the fact that he isn't going to drink tonight because he's with me. But it's not worth it to me to feel "in" and do all that stuff. I'd rather feel left out.

When I tried to find out what's really inside them, these college kids seemed so shallow. They were more grown-up than high school kids. They had a major. They had to worry about a job, a living, a place to live, and their parents getting older and stuff like that; but they were still really caught up in something I thought was junior high stuff. My priorities have changed in that I'm trying to make major things major and minor things minor. They're worried about what they'll wear, what they're going to do this weekend . . . things that don't really matter.

I think things out more now. I can't afford to make any major dumb mistakes about my life. I have a strong belief in positive attitude. You can't talk about odds because everybody dies. Period. The odds are those: They die. How soon, of course, is another question.

When the doctor told me that I didn't have to take medicine anymore, that I was cured, I said to myself, "Okay, he says I'm cured. He should know. But I might get sick again."

I wanted to tell everybody that the doctor said I was cured, but I hesitated. As far as I know, they have no cure. I think the only cure, really, is time. I look at it this way: If you can have *some* time, then if you get sick, good grief, who cares? You had such a good time while you were well. Now if *that's* cured, that's all right with me.

Linda Von Seggers

Soft-spoken but full of sparkle, Linda Von Seggers abides by a single rule: Stay with it. When she was slapped down with leukemia in 1972, her family had just sold their home in Michigan and moved to Florida, fulfilling lifelong plans to buy their own business. But cancer foreclosed on their dream. They had no medical insurance for Linda.

Her tight-knit family vowed to be honest with themselves. Among house rules, they outlawed whispering about Linda and insisted that their everyday routine be maintained as much as possible. Simply, they let Linda know that "they expected me to recover."

I was fourteen when I was diagnosed with leukemia. I'm nineteen now. I've been in remission five years. I've been lucky.

When we found out, all I knew about leukemia was that it's a blood disorder. The only experience I'd had with it was a little girl we knew who had leukemia and who, over a year, became really sick and died. So that was the first thing I thought of: When you get leukemia, you die.

But I never really thought I was going to die. I just couldn't imagine it. I think that may be why I was able to keep a positive attitude. I never really thought about it that much.

Even though I was sick, I never realized how bad off I was. Maybe my parents did, but I didn't.

At fourteen, I was kind of chubby. I weighed 130. But I lost twenty-six pounds in one week. That's how sick I was. I had temperatures of 104 degrees all day and all night, day after day until finally they just sent me home. I think they thought I might feel better at home.

I couldn't wait. I wanted to show everybody how great I looked without that weight. At least I thought I looked great. I never saw what I really looked like. I could just see that weight going off.

It took a long time for me to realize I had anything serious. Even after they did the bone marrow test, I didn't think about it being anything.

The doctor made a point of explaining the steps I would go through in reacting. You know, Phase One: Why me? and all that. He was right. But even as they were telling me what would happen, I was telling myself, "That's not going to happen to me. Not me."

Sometimes I'd wonder if the drugs really were going to help me. But I did research papers on cancer drugs for biology and English courses, and that helped. I felt reassured reading about the drugs in magazine articles. I checked out the different side effects and statistics on remissions, and it made me feel more secure knowing the drugs had been successful with other cases.

The doctor also talked to me about the medication. I always knew I had to take it. But there were times when I was ready to give up. Then I'd think about a guy living down the street from me who was born with an open spine. He had to go through so many operations that I could look at him and say to myself, "Look at him. What am I worrying about?"

When I first got sick I had a boy friend. But the whole time I was in the hospital he never sent me one card. Never called. I thought, "What's wrong?"

When I got home I kept asking my friends why he never called me or anything. Finally they broke down and told me,

"He said he didn't want a girl friend who was only going to live three months, who had leukemia."

And I said, "Well, what is he talking about? I'm living longer than three months."

That kind of gave me a little push, too, because I thought, "I'm gonna show him."

At first I wanted to stay in bed all the time. I was pretty weak, but I would probably still be in bed if it weren't for my parents and friends. I have a couple of friends who used to come every day and say, "Now come on, Linda, get up," and they'd make me get up and walk around a little bit.

And then they went out and fixed up my bicycle. It sat out on the carport for a long time, but finally one day they said, "This is it. You're going out there, and you're going to start exercising."

And then they came over and planted a little flower garden in the backyard so I could go outside and take care of the flowers. Oh, that was a big help, yes! I had to keep going for my friends.

I felt sorry for myself a lot. I think there again my parents and my friends helped tremendously. They knew when I was feeling sorry for myself. It's a matter of positive outlook, keeping the faith, constantly looking ahead and thinking things are going to be a lot better.

There were times when I got really down when it didn't matter how much I tried to bring myself up or how much my friends tried, I still felt bad.

Everybody else would be going out, and I couldn't go out. And I would think, "It's not fair. Why me? Why did I have to get sick? There are so many people—murderers and thieves and crooks—people really doing bad things. Why couldn't it happen to them?"

But as time went on I learned so much. I've had so many experiences that when I think about it I'm kind of glad. Even though I had some pain, I'm kind of glad. I'm special. I have a teacher who's surviving on only half a lung. Just barely making it. And she used to say, "Linda, it's not bad that you have it. Only special people have things like this. You learn a lot from it." I really have.

I used to just want to stay in my room and listen to my stereo. I wanted everybody to just leave me alone, bring me my food when I needed to eat and that would be it. But once I started getting out again I saw a lot of things that I hadn't seen before. The more I did, the more I wanted to do. It built up.

When I went back to school I looked different. People didn't recognize me. I wore my wig the first day I went back. It was a long shag, and I was a lot thinner. I looked better than before, really. I was sitting on a bench when I heard some guy say, "Whoa, who's that?"

Altogether, I lost my hair three times. The first time with radiation. I had long blond hair. It was a bad experience, but I think part of that is because you worry about it more than other people do.

I thought when I went back to school everybody would make fun of me. They accepted it. They even made jokes like, "Hey, here comes Kojak." People thought that was cruel, but it helped. Joking around about it kept it in the open. Attitude made a big difference.

The doctors told me long beforehand that my hair would fall out, so I had time to think about it. They said after I'd had radiation three or four times, it would start thinning out. I didn't believe it. My hair never fell out when I had vincristine, and they always told me it was going to.

I did finally accept the fact that it was going to come out one day, and you just had to do the best you could.

If you know you'll lose your hair, I'd say go ahead early, before your hair falls out, and try to get a wig as close to your hair as possible. Many people won't even notice you're wearing a wig. You can get them to shape the wig and make it look very much like your own hair.

The most upsetting part of going bald was actually seeing the hair fall out. My grandmother was staying at our house the day it came out. She used to love my long hair, and she had decided to brush it for me. That's when it all came out. She just kept on brushing and brushing, and she cried and cried and cried. It really upset me. It wasn't so much that my hair was falling out, but that she was so upset about it. And the fact that it came out in one big clump, all at once, was a big shock.

At first I wore the wig, but it was so itchy I decided to go without it. I wore a scarf all the time. I had one tiny clump of hair right in front, and I used to drape it across my forehead and wear it that way. I thought I was fooling everyone. Now that I think about it—when you look at the other bald kids at the hospital—you can see that there isn't any hair back there under that scarf, but I never thought about that.

Once I started wearing a scarf to school, a lot of other people did. I think maybe they wanted to make me feel a little better. I don't think it was because it looked really nice.

It took about eight months for it to grow. It was like a super-short pixie. The first time it came in really thin and straight. Then it fell out again, which really didn't matter because it was so short anyway.

Then it came back in wavy and nice, then thinned out again after I had large doses of cytoxan.

After that it grew back and stayed. It was still super short when I stopped wearing my scarf, but my mother convinced me that if I stopped wearing my scarf it would grow out better. She was right. But I thought it was way too short.

Everywhere I'd go, people would say, "Where did you get your hair cut?"

I'd say, "You don't want one. It's the most expensive haircut you can get."

I was worrying about the money situation. When I was diagnosed, we had just sold the house in Michigan and my father was going to use all the money to start his own business in Florida. I didn't have any insurance, so the medical expenses went through the money from the house just like that. I used to tell my mother I felt bad about it and everything, but she said it didn't matter. Any amount of money. Just to keep on going.

When I did think about my own death, I always wondered what it would do to everybody else. How they would feel.

When people come up and say, "Wow, you're doing *so* good, you're just like a miracle," it builds you up even more. They're hoping for you, too. It makes you believe they expect you to recover. You can tell which people are thinking, "Poor kid, she's only got a few more months." That really makes you feel rotten.

My mother's friends would often come over, and they would start whispering, and she'd say, "Stop whispering. We're going to talk about it openly, and Linda can hear everything we're saying. If you talk about her sickness behind her back, she's going to think it's worse than it really is." So we always had open conversations, and with my friends I was always really happy to explain anything to them. I just wanted to let them know that I wasn't doing terrible. A lot of times I had to convince people that I wasn't as bad off as they thought I was.

And many times, even though I was sick as a dog, I'd take my little pan, even though I was constantly vomiting, and go to school. They knew I was really sick but they still let me go to school. I think staying around people helps keep your spirits up.

Even though my teachers came to the house, I still went to school and had lunch with the kids. I used to go to all four lunch hours. I think it's great to keep the activity going and to live as normal a life as possible.

Some of my friends, however, thought cancer was contagious. I went back to class, and a couple of girls didn't want to sit by me. But I didn't know anything about cancer either until I got it, so I just said, "But you're not going to get it. It's not contagious."

The teacher talked to them. Everybody talked it out and finally came to the conclusion that it was all right to sit by me. A lot of times in my classes people were really curious about it, so we'd talk about it. That made it much easier for me because then they knew a little more about what I was going through.

In fact, some friends got so overprotective it was very frustrating. Everyone would be outside walking around barefoot, and I'd take off my shoes and right away somebody would say, "Oh, put your shoes back on." And at dances people would say, "Okay, Linda, you'd better sit down. You're gonna overdo." I wanted to be like everybody else so much. I didn't want them to treat me any differently. Every now and then I would want to do something impulsive just to say, "See?"

I used to take my friends up to the hospital with me. It's a great idea, but I haven't seen many other people bringing their friends up much. Not even brothers and sisters.

I've done it all the way through junior high, high school, and college. I'd bring my boy friends up so they could see because they would often wonder, you know. It helps. They knew. They watched.

My doctor would put them to work. He would have them hold the cotton when he was taking out an IV. They kind of got involved with everything, which helps out tremendously.

The principal at school would let me sign out so many kids to take with me. I usually brought two or three. And we'd all pile up together with my parents in a hotel room and have a great time. I think it gave them a feeling of being needed.

Going in for a bone marrow now, after five years, is more

upsetting than it was at first. When you go for months and months and months without one and then have to go in, it's hard. I'll go in the bathroom and get all the crying done first. I think it puts the doctors more at ease the calmer you are. It helps to talk to them the whole time. The more relaxed the atmosphere, the better it goes.

I don't think you should hold it all inside yourself. That just makes it worse. When I talk to other kids with cancer who are feeling down, I tell them it may be painful sometimes, but it's not as bad as you think. When I look back on it now, everything went pretty fast. Anything the doctors had to do they'd do in a hurry. You just have to live with it.

Cheryl Hall

When Cheryl Hall was diagnosed with cancer, her doctors told her flatly, "We think you'll die."

Wide-eyed and full of indignation, Cheryl picked up a roll of tape, threw it at them, and said, "Are you God? You can't tell me I'll die."

For nearly two years she fought with quiet faith. As she said, "When I first started out, I had a lot of courage. Everybody commented about that. But it slowly dwindles. I've learned that when they're going to do something more to you, you can't pray, 'God, don't let them hurt me.' You have to pray for the strength to cope with it."

On March 1, 1979, Cheryl died. She was fifteen. Here's her story, in her own words.

I've always said, "I'm going to write a book one day, and it's going to be about me." I've read all these cancer books, but they put me into tears because the persons dies. This one would be different because I'm still alive. They can read about something that was good. They say all these people that died, they were such heroes. But who wants to read about somebody who's dead? What good is it gonna do?

It started in June, right after we got out of school. I woke up one morning, and I didn't feel so hot. I felt like maybe I was catching a cold.

And so you do all the usual things: You take aspirin and drink lots of orange juice. I did that, and I felt better for about two weeks. Then I woke up again feeling rotten.

I drug around for two weeks until my mom finally took me to the doctor. He looked at me and decided it was probably a virus. He said I just had to wear it out.

So we went home and started the medicine he'd given us. I was feeling well enough to go with my mom and sister up to Indiana to see my grandmother. It took about three days driving from Clearwater (Florida).

When we got there I was feeling pretty bad. I was throwing up everything I ate and having hot flashes and feeling faint. And I was starting to have problems breathing.

I was also losing weight. I weighed 130 pounds, and I was really glad in a way that my appetite was gone. Before, I'd look at other people and wonder how they stayed so skinny. I really liked to eat, and I was trying everything to lose weight. And all of a sudden I was really losing.

But my mom was getting worried.

When we got home she took me back to the doctor, but he said I just hadn't worn the virus out yet. A couple of days later I was having such a hard time breathing that I was bent forward over a pillow and coughing all this stuff up. It was a constant cough. I couldn't stop. Couldn't hold down any food. I was thirsty a lot, and I just didn't feel like doing anything.

The morning I went to the doctor I was feeling really bad. My color was sallow because I hadn't gotten enough oxygen. I was hyperventilated, breathing through my stomach, which is like swelling.

When they pushed on my leg there was a dent where he put his finger. So he thought maybe it was hyperthyroidism. Like all I'd have to do is go to the hospital, get lab work every week, and take pills. So I wasn't really worried. Cancer was the farthest thing from my mind.

I had never been seriously sick before. I got a lot of colds, but I was otherwise pretty healthy. Nobody in our family has ever had any serious illnesses.

The doctor sent me to the hospital and put us in a room, and then he came in and did some lab work—blood tests. When they drew my blood it was purple because I lacked so much oxygen.

Then they did what's called a thoracentesis (say thora-sin-TEA-sis), where they go in and draw out fluids out of your chest, fluids that have accumulated in the lungs.

When they took an X ray of my lungs, they saw three puddles. They were going to go in there and draw it out, but when he was in there poking around he said he felt something in there that didn't belong.

He told my mom that, and later, when I came home from the big ordeal the first time around, she said that when he said he felt something she knew something was really wrong. You know, you get the feeling sometimes that something's going to happen.

Pretty soon it got so bad they were giving me a nasal cannula for oxygen. I was pretty wide awake. It was uncomfortable. My nose was sore and it dried it out and when I ate I got a lot of air bubbles in my stomach. But after a while I got very dependent on it. I was getting progressively worse. Finally they put me in this special care unit for children. It was all decorated with horses on the drapes and all that, and they did two biopsies. I was really sick by then.

They just inserted a needle and took some tissue out, and then they inserted two chest tubes and took out fluid.

On my side, I have little round scars from it. They numbed it and all I could feel was a lot of pushing and pressure. I couldn't roll around and that really drove me nuts, because I like to move around a lot when I'm in bed.

During that time, I daydreamed about what it would be like when I went home. How it would be different. My mom and dad were remodeling our house. I expected it to be like having my birthday every day because of all the attention. My grandparents and an aunt were at home, too, helping out.

At the hospital, they had a suction machine going day and night to get all the fluid out, and I was on oxygen. They hadn't diagnosed it yet. They finally diagnosed it as neuroblastoma: tumors.

When I was in the intensive care unit there were a lot of babies brought in that would die. It would really shake you up because you'd say, "I wonder if this is what always happens. I wonder if this is why they put me here."

But I decided the babies just lay there and can't do anything. They don't know how to fight.

I was there for about a week when they finally came in and one doctor told me there was nothing they could do.

They said that all they could do was put me in a room and keep me comfortable. The doctor told me flat out, "We think you're going to die."

That really made me mad. The doctor was acting as though if he couldn't help me nobody could.

It was unbelievable. I'm ashamed to say it, but I picked up a roll of tape and threw it at him. I yelled, "Are you God? You can't tell me I'm going to die." From that point on, I said, "I'm not going to."

But I knew that what I had could kill you, and I was really scared. In a way I felt like I was going against God to fight. Like maybe God wanted me to die. When I'd see a baby die, I would try to remember there's a reason He let it die. Maybe God was testing my faith.

Intensive care was really pretty bad. I was conscious most of the time. In fact, I don't think I slept a wink the whole time. I was in a bed under the light, and I was very wide awake.

All I could eat were orange Popsicles. Every now and then they'd sit me up in a chair, and I'd be humped over a pillow when the doctor came in. He'd ask how I was. I'd go, "I'm fine, I'm fine." No matter how bad I felt I'd always say I felt fine. I just never like to complain. It really made me feel better if I said that.

Pretty soon I was too sick to even sit up in a chair. I wasn't in pain, but I was really sick. I had a mask over my nose and mouth with mist in it you breathe to loosen your lungs and give them elasticity.

The tumor was pressing against nerves and making me really hoarse. It was growing very fast. They could watch it grow. They showed my dad the scan, and he traced it on my chest for me. It covered my whole chest down to my waist.

They had taken me out of intensive care. But my family doctor got on the phone at three in the morning and started calling hospitals all over the country—New York, Houston, Miami, Gainesville—trying to find somebody who could help me.

He found a doctor in Gainesville who was studying neuroblastoma and having some success. He talked to that doctor, who said, "Bring her here. I really want to see her."

To get me from Clearwater to Gainesville, they had the option of taking me up in a jet ambulance or the back seat of my dad's car or in a regular ambulance. The jet ambulance was out because it would take a lot of money, and then they have trouble with oxygen and people not being able to breathe. The back seat of my dad's car was kind of out, too, because they would have had to have a nurse or somebody back there, and my dad didn't want to do it. So they put me in an out-of-town ambulance. But half way up the road the ambulance broke down. My mom said it was one of the scariest parts in the whole time because the oxygen cut off, and I was gasping. At that time if somebody took that oxygen away for good, I don't think I would have made it. It's like being hooked on drugs. You just have to have it. I had to have air conditioning, too. I couldn't stand the hot weather, and this was in the summer.

So they called another ambulance to hurry up and come get me. Then they turned on the oxygen, and everybody was really relieved. So we got halfway down I-75 and started to run out of gas. I'll never forget it.

There were two ambulance drivers in the front and my mom and a woman paramedic in the back. She was taking blood pressure, respiration, stuff like that. They stopped at a truck stop, and they went in and bought me three candy bars, a bag of Fritos, and orange pop.

When you see an ambulance going down the road you expect to see a person laying out in the back. But here I was, sitting up eating all this food!

When we got to Shands Teaching Hospital, the atmosphere was so different. At my local hospital they worry more about paperwork, more about appearances, more about the way they look to other people than they do about the people inside and saving lives. Whereas at Shands they seem kind of disorganized, but they're more worried about saving the patient's life. When we got in the emergency room, my mom was praying. She thought, "Oh, what have we done? We've made an awful mistake."

They took me up to a room and started an IV—the first one I'd ever had—and put in an arterial line. They had taken out the chest tubes and stitched up the holes. So Doctor Barbosa came in and said he wanted to start some doses of cytoxan and vincristine because he's had luck before using those drugs. He's very aggressive with the drugs. I was getting bigger doses than most people get.

When I first started I had a lot of courage. Everybody commented on that. But it slowly dwindled. If I had to have a chest tube now, I'm afraid I'd get up and run, because I know what it's like.

The chemotherapy started working as soon as it was in

there. After about three months the tumor had shrunk enough for surgery. They were ecstatic. They said my case was just unbelievable.

The night before surgery the whole team came in and told me what they were going to be doing. They were going to try to get as much tumor as they could. It was a combination of removing the tumor and exploring. They didn't really know what was going on in there. I'd seen all the X rays. You wouldn't believe the difference in them.

Surgery seemed so straightforward. I was feeling I might get rid of it once and for all. I thought I might not need any more chemotherapy, ever.

But they thought they might have to do a mastectomy. I was fourteen, and that was a big shock. I don't know how I would have handled it. They didn't know how much they were going to get or whether they were going to get any at all, if the surgery would be just opening me up and sewing me up again. He said he might have to rearrange stuff in there, put in some artificial tissue, take out the whole lung, take out part of the lung—they just didn't know. They couldn't promise me anything.

I didn't get really scared until they told me about the mastectomy, and then about the tubes I was probably going to have.

I was going to have an airway, which scared me the worst because I was afraid I was going to wake up with the thing down my throat. I was going to have a gastro-intestinal tube that goes down your nose into your stomach. I was going to have a tube in my bladder, two chest tubes, an arterial line, an IV and another IV for blood. That's eight tubes. It was just plain scary because I thought I was going to be like Frankenstein, that lightning would activate me.

My mom and I did a lot of crying together when nobody else was there. We kind of sat and cried for a little bit. Everybody does. It's natural. I said my prayers in the morning and got up and had to take a bath in a surgical scrub that turns everything yellow, and then I had to take my nail polish off and then they gave me a shot of morphine, which really konks you out.

When we went in the elevator I could tell my mom was scared. I was in surgery for five hours. Anyway, when I got down in the recovery room I didn't feel as though time had passed. I hadn't dreamed. It was as if I weren't there at all. It was like I wasn't asleep, but by the time I was awake enough to comprehend, the trachea tube was out and the bladder tube was out and I was breathing on my own.

My mom and dad came in, and when I saw that I was laying there alive, I felt really safe. It was a time of contentment, one of the times I was really at peace. I just felt as if I could let the world be and go to sleep.

When I'm in the hospital I just can't be at ease sleeping. It's a very insecure feeling. You never know when somebody's going to come in and poke you.

After surgery I had a lot of pain. They get you sitting up right away so you don't get pneumonia. When I would sit up, I would cry because it hurt so bad.

Every night they came in and gave me a shot of morphine to put me to sleep. You feel really good for a little bit and then you go to sleep. You wake up and you have the worst hangover in the world. You just go through the same thing day after day.

About that time I started getting mail from my friends. That was great. I just loved it.

Then one day the doctors came in and explained it to my parents and me. They said they got most of the cancer, but that I would need more chemotherapy. Earlier, my dad had had a heart-to-heart talk with one of the students who was in there watching when Dr. Rodgers did it, and he said he was absolutely magnificent. He said a regular surgeon would have gone in there, looked at it, and closed me back up.

But this doctor went in there and knew when they were going to get into trouble and took precautions, and they got about ninety percent of it. About ten percent of it was around main arteries, and they didn't want to mess with that.

The pain afterwards was unbelievable. The last three days in the hospital were spent getting chemotherapy. It was what I call the tough stuff: cytoxan and vincristine. They give you this combination first thing in the morning, dripping it into you every two hours all day, so that by dark you're not so sick that you can't go to sleep.

I had to have a catheter, which I really hate, because the chemotherapy was so toxic they don't want it to lay in your bladder. So they irrigate your bladder to keep it from becoming irritated by the cytoxan.

So I went home feeling really sore and sick. Among other things, I became much more sensitive to noise, and the taste of milk seemed funny to me.

The day after I got home, I had to go back for radiation therapy. I took that for nine weeks. We commuted between home and the hospital every other day.

Radiation therapy doesn't hurt at all. It gives you a nice tan on your chest and your back.

Most of my teachers were understanding, to a point. Some were downright sarcastic. One assigned me a whole pile of homework, and I said, "Well, I might not be able to get all this done right away."

It wasn't that I couldn't do the work. But I had different priorities. I had to work on staying alive. I couldn't work on getting straight A's on my report card.

One day I came home from school crying. One of my girl friends was going to throw a party, and the girls were supposed to ask the boys. And I asked one, and he said, "Yeah, sure."

So we had a party on the last day of school, and he said, "Do you mind if I don't go?"

And I said, "No, that's okay."

So I went back in the corner, and I just broke down. And my friend came over, and she said, "What's wrong?" I told her what he said, and she said, "Well, I'll go find out."

She went over and talked to him, and she found out that he was really kind of scared of me.

I went home and talked to my mom, and she said, "You know, when people don't understand they don't know what to make of it. They think it's worse than it really is."

My hair thinned out when I had my first chemotherapy. But I wasn't really bald for about half a year later. Losing it was like shedding. I used to sleep with a stocking cap on my head because I got so cold.

I remember especially waking up on Christmas Eve morning with a big bald spot in the middle of my head. There were all these little hairs lying on the pillow. I said, "Mom, I have to go and get my wig trimmed. Come here and look!" She came in, and we both laughed so hard because it looked so funny.

I was just glad I was there and alive.

I wish everybody knew as much about cancer as I do now. I think I've changed a lot of people's perspective about the word "cancer." When I used to hear the word I shuddered. I'd think "death" right away. I know I changed one medical student's idea. He thought on the cancer ward everybody was going to be dying.

There were things my doctors knew I shouldn't do but that I wanted to do. There were a lot of times when my blood was low when the doctor didn't want me in the swimming pool. You know, I might catch pneumonia. But a lot of times I went to school anyway. I went to the movies anyway. I did everything, no matter what my blood was like.

The doctor told my mom she'd done me a real favor. She hadn't crippled my mind. She never made me think I wasn't worth anything anymore because this had happened to me. It's all in the way you think.

You have to be really positive. You have to be really aggressive and courageous. You've got to be downright mean about it. You just have to say, "It won't beat me."

We've had to do without a lot of things because of medical expenses. It has strained my family. They probably snap at each other a little bit more. They're a little bit more tense sometimes. It makes me feel bad, but I can't blame myself. How much do you think your family values you? You think your mother would rather have the money in her pocket than have you? It's hard to think that's true.

I think it has been a lot harder on my parents than on me. My parents had to stay there and watch me, but they couldn't fight for me. I'm sure that made it really hard. All you can do is tell them you're not going to give up.

One thing I really regret is that nobody told my little sister what was going on. She was only eleven at the time. She was really scared. With little kids, they imagine things bad based on what you tell them.

She's still kind of mad because nobody told her. In a way, she's a little hurt. Grandma and Grandpa were in the house, and Mom and Dad and my aunt. And she didn't know why everybody was crying, or why everybody was so sad, why she had to keep going to the neighbor's house and spending the night.

It made her scared. And nobody would tell her. In fact, I think I'm the first one who told her. She was talking about what they do at the hospital, and I said, "Do you know what's wrong with me?"

And she said, "No."

And I told her that I had a tumor and that it was cancerous. She goes, "Really?"

And I said, "Nobody ever told you that?"

And she said, "No."

And that really made me mad because I felt she had a right to know.

You wouldn't believe how stories change when kids tell them, because everybody in the neighborhood and everybody at school had different ideas. Everyone thought I had a tumor anywhere from my big toe to my brain.

They all knew I was really sick, and they helped out a lot. The kids were usually better about it than the adults. The ones my own age seemed to understand what I was going through.

Now we don't worry about anything. Somehow everything is going to work out. Many things people get all upset about seem so stupid to me. Such little things. If you're standing there alive, you've got the grass below your feet and the sun above your head, what can you worry about? Worry is a waste of time. It really is.

I'm a lot more relaxed now.

Sometimes it seems like only nice people get cancer. I asked "Why me?" millions and millions and millions of times. Lots of friends smoke cigarettes, they lie to their parents, they get into a lot of trouble. So why me? I guess it is because I was strong enough to handle it, and they weren't. I appreciate life so much more now. I'm a better person for having it.

Alice Demick

She calls herself a people pleaser. Trademark? A sense of joy that never runs dry. When her friends signed her high school yearbook, they wrote the same simple tribute in a hundred different ways: "Alice, we know you by your smile."

Month after month for years, Alice Demick lived with pain. She took prednisone seven days a week, had transfusions every four days, and finally at nineteen, faced the grim odds of a bone marrow transplant.

The youngest of nine children, and without a father, Alice worked after school to help pay the insurmountable medical bills her family bore because she had aplastic anemia. Now twenty, successful and single, Alice lives—for the first time in fourteen years—as a healthy person. In addition, she attends college two nights a week near her hometown of Freeburg, Illinois.

I have aplastic anemia. In simple language that means I have an inadequate number of different kinds of blood cells. It's like a building that has a block missing. That one missing piece doesn't build any blood like the other bricks, so you have to have transfusions.

With aplastic anemia, you gets lots of bruises, which are really another form of bleeding—bleeding under the skin—and that uses up blood. But your body doesn't replace it like it normally would.

People with aplastic anemia have trouble breathing. When they try to walk with somebody their own age, at the same pace, they can't do it. They just can't do it. It's an awful feeling.

I was in third grade when I was diagnosed with aplastic. I spent my ninth birthday in the hospital. My mother doesn't drive, but every day—for ninety-eight days—she had someone drive her to the hospital. It was an hour there and an hour back.

I didn't know it at the time, but they told her there was no hope. They had no cures. But they put me on prednisone. I took thirty-one pills a day. I remember when I finally came home from the hospital I weighed ninety-eight pounds. A nine-year-old! I was huge. My older brother and his friends thought I was so cute because I looked like a little balloon: big cheeks, pudgy, just really blown up.

On prednisone, I pretty well stabilized. Until eighth grade I was in a kind of remission. Then I started menstruating.

I never had platelets over twelve thousand (normal is two hundred thousand to three hundred thousand). When I began menstruating, I hemorrhaged. I had to have transfusions two times a week. In the beginning I didn't have much trouble with that, but the longer I had the transfusions the worse it got: chills, fever, headaches, and always the risk that I would get hepatitis (which I did later get).

I was on prednisone nine years. It affected me in many ways. I remember prednisone caused nightmares. Some people hallucinate on prednisone. I had the same nightmare over and over again. I dreamed these people had balls on long chains and they were beating my mother and me. Those kinds of dreams.

I always worried about how I looked. Prednisone caused what they call an "elephant hump" on the back of my neck. It wasn't that noticeable, but *I* knew it was there. I'd have hair way down on the back of my neck. The drug also made my hair very thick. Hair grew on my face, and oh, I used to hate that! I got my pubic hair when I was nine years old, and I was embarrassed about that, too. I felt like I couldn't face anyone anymore. Then my doctor sent me to another doctor—not a pediatrician—because I had this pubic hair, and that was a real rejection for me and hard to take.

As I got older, I always felt that I never got asked out because I was so fat. Who would want to go out with a fat girl? I felt left out. I thought it was all because I was sick. That was a big thing I blamed on being sick. I never went to a prom. It was all I could do to walk two blocks.

But later, after I recovered, I found that if you continually miss it, you're never going to be content. I think I'm over the period when you continually say to yourself, "I missed this," and "I didn't get to do that," or "I've got to make up for things I never did before." I've found that a lot of the things I imagined were so great aren't the way I pictured them. Some things are a big disappointment. But I didn't know that then.

I hemorrhaged the whole summer of eighth grade. Once, I got something caught in my throat and I began coughing, and my whole face turned black and blue, just from coughing.

From eighth grade through my senior year in high school, I had blood transfusions weekly and sometimes twice a week. Two pints. I pushed myself a lot, and I think that's good. I worked at the library after school. I always felt like I had to go. I just had to. Something just said to me, "Keep going." And then I'd go home and maybe sleep for a couple hours, between work and supper.

As it kept going, I kept getting more reactions to the transfusions. Finally, in 1976, I was told that unless I had a bone marrow transplant, I would die. Even with the bone marrow transplant my chances were fifty-fifty. It was life or death.

When I was younger I really hadn't thought about dying. I

didn't think about it until it came right down to it. The week before I had to go to Seattle for the transplant, I thought about it a lot.

This is the thing: People who aren't terminally ill don't really think about it. They may say to themselves, "Oh, I'm going to die someday. So what? Big deal. I might be fifty-four. I might be eighty-two." But when you are a teenager and told that you might die soon, you're going to have to think about death and how you want your life to be *now*. Maybe you won't be here to make it that way later on.

You don't think about a career. A career is just out of the picture. You live one day to the next, and you make *that* day the best. And you try not to regret any day you live.

When they told me I would have to go to Seattle, right after I heard the news I went over to my friend Pam's house; and Pam and I went up to her room, and we both started crying. We were scared. You need somebody like that to cry to. We thought this might be it. We talked about it for a long time.

I think teenagers need somebody who will listen to them. Even if it's somebody who doesn't understand what it's like to have cancer. If they'll just *try* to understand. Knowing that they'll come, at any time of the day or night, can be very consoling. Not a family member. You need somebody outside the family who you can show your emotions to, rattle on and on and on, or cry to if you want to cry, or scream if you want to scream.

When somebody close—your family—has to go through all the agony and worry over whether you're going to die, you feel guilty. You don't want to put them through any more by crying or telling them you're afraid. It's hard. It takes courage all the way down. Your brothers and sisters get neglected, and they tease you and call you a baby and tell you that if it weren't for you, Mom wouldn't have to go through all this.

People have different ways of coping. Some people can't cope. They just block it out. Just say, "It's not there. Forget it. It's not there."

Those people are a little unfortunate because they don't bring themselves to reality. I think coping is just realizing it and doing the best with it . . . just facing the fact that you have this thing and you might die from it.

What about little kids? They cry. That's *their* bravery. They cry.

When I was sick, I could never bring myself to cry publicly. I could *not* do it. It just was not part of me. I could cry at home, but I could never cry in a hospital.

I remember the first time I cried in front of a nurse. It was when I had bleeding muscles. And afterwards I felt ashamed. But then I realized you have to cry sometimes. Why not cry? Some people need to cry in front of people to get sympathy or to get somebody to console them. Me, I'm embarrassed when I cry.

But I think people should be able to cry. If it hurts, cry. Don't think you're making the nurse or the doctor feel bad. That's what I did. I couldn't make anybody feel bad. I think that's why I always held the tears back.

There's a kind of aloneness that comes with sickness. You just feel lonely. Desolate, at times.

When I came home from Seattle all my friends had gone off to college. I thought, "Where are all my friends? This is not the place I left." I got really depressed. It seemed as though nobody was there. Brothers and sisters helped. True friends helped. If you're down, they'll come pick you up.

Then circumstances, like a job, maybe going back to school . . . I began making afghans, and people even bought some of them. And I did some typing at home for the library. Catalog cards. That really helped.

Once you've been sick, I find that decisions are much

harder to make. You think things out. I think that may stem from the fact that when you're sick, you're catered to. Maybe not outright, but you *are* sheltered. You don't have a lot of the decisions that teens have to make right away. As far as going out for track, say, those kinds of choices are already made. You know you have to go to the doctor once a week. It becomes a routine, a part of your living. Once you get into the hang of it and get to know people at the hospital and talk to people about it, you accept the fact that you have to live your life the way it is.

I think a lot of teenagers who get sick as teens have a hard time at first. But most teens are adult enough.

They can't just rush it into a few minutes. It's going to take a long talk, but eventually they're going to realize it's not so bad. I feel like a very fortunate person. I think everybody is, if they just look at it in comparison to other people.

There is a child abuse center down the hall from our clinic, and when you see the kids they bring in there, you realize that mental brutality can be much worse than physical brutality. My experiences were very good mentally. I'm rich in experiences. Sickness really is a blessing, believe it or not. You grow so much. You cope with it. You learn how to cope.

Steve Bennett

Plenty of times, Steve Bennett, fifteen, wanted to run. Run until every football coach in the country stood up and cheered. Run until no hint of cancer, no chemotherapy could touch him. But Steve didn't run. He sat down and learned to take it.

From a family of football heroes, Steve was number three in line and already bragging about what he would become when, in 1977, osteogenic sarcoma changed the score. Doctors amputated his leg at the hip. Eight months later, cancer slammed back into his life, this time in his lung.

Two years into treatment, Steve speaks with quiet understanding. "It isn't going to be easy for me," he says, then adds, "but then, nothing's easy."

I came into the hospital about a year ago for what I thought was a sore muscle in my knee. They came in and took X rays and wanted to do a biopsy. They found out it was bone cancer. When they came to tell me, I thought they were going to tell me when I could go home. But it was a whole different thing.

At first I didn't know what bone cancer was. I knew what cancer was. They told me they were going to amputate. I thought they were going to amputate to my knee. Then they told me they were going to have to amputate all the way up. I just couldn't believe it.

I was in football then, and that was what my career was going to be. It just took me a while to accept it. At first I didn't want to do it. But then I got to thinking, "What's more important, football or your life?" Football isn't that important. I made up my mind I was going to let them do it, and I wasn't going to be moping around all the time. I made up my mind that I was going to live. Just because my leg's gone doesn't mean I'm going to be better or worse than anybody else. I just made up my mind I was going to be happy.

At first they told me by myself. Then they asked me if I wanted my parents there, and I said, "Yeah." And my brothers and sisters came in, and we talked.

My dad really helped me. He told me people respect somebody who gets down to the problem and really solves it, somebody who gets over obstacles in their lives. He told me he'd be with me through it and that he loved me and that everything would be all right.

When they did the biopsy, it only took them about ten minutes before they knew it was cancer, but they asked my mom if she wanted them to wait and let me know or go ahead and amputate.

She said, "No, wait, and let him know."

I'm glad they did that. I don't know what I'd do if I woke up and was without a leg. I think when they tell you it gives you a chance to be prepared. Sort of a last good-bye thing.

The day they told me, I took a long look at my right toes and moved them around. My leg was in a cast, but that night I didn't call for a pain pill. I wanted to feel it. I was glad it was there.

After the surgery I stayed in the hospital about two weeks. Then the doctors started talking to me about chemotherapy, follow-up drugs. They said they were going to start me on methotrexate. I didn't think it was anything, really. He said there'd be a little nausea, my hair might fall out. But with methotrexate my hair didn't fall out. About six months into chemotherapy I started taking Adriamycin, and that got my hair. I think it was harder to accept my hair falling out than losing my leg.

But I got a cap and a wig. I told everybody it was a wig because I could just see somebody coming down the hall and snatching the hat. I guess I had a complex about my hair.

I'm still wearing a wig when I'm around my friends, but when I come out of town, to the hospital, I go without it. My hair came in a different color, darker, and it was curly.

Adriamycin is one drug I just hate. It makes you sick for about two days, and then you have to go back the next day and take it, and take it again, and that makes you sick more. When I first took Adriamycin, the doctor said it would be about two weeks before my hair would come out. And two weeks came, then two and a half, and I had pretty high hopes it wouldn't come out. But then one night when I was ready for bed it felt like pins sticking in my scalp, and when I scratched it I had a handful of hair.

We had the address of some people who would match your hair perfectly with a wig, so we sent them a picture and some hair and they did it. A really good looking wig. But it looked fake up here at the crown. So I'd stick a hat on it and you couldn't tell.

When you take the Adriamycin you vomit right then because a taste comes in your mouth. Some people don't believe that, but it does. A taste comes in your mouth. It makes you want to throw up. So you do. It lasts for about a day. The next morning you feel terrible, but you have to go take it again. That's the hard part. Just to force yourself to take it again. I just say, "Let's get this over with."

They found something on my lung. They thought it was a blood vessel at first. But they did a scan and decided they'd better go in and take it out, and it was cancer. They took it out and took a little of my lung out. After that they put me on methotrexate for two years.

When they told me I was going to have to come in every two weeks for two years, at first I said, "No." I told them I wouldn't do it. You get frustrated and jealous and mad at the world. You get tired of it. That's what is really rotten. That's why I said no to that first medicine. I was tired. I was tired of having to go to the hospital. It just made me sick to go into the hospital. I lost a lot of weight. Gained it back after the surgery on my leg. I was pretty well as big as the other boys, but after they put me back on those treatments I lost all my weight and went down to skin and bones.

I thought the drugs that they'd given to me before had been a waste—a waste of time. You know, I always thought, "What if these drugs don't work? What if I'm going through all this for nothing?" I told myself, "If they find some more cancer on me while I'm taking these drugs, then I won't take it any more." But my dad talked me into it.

He taught me this rhyme: "A quitter never wins, a winner never quits." In order to live I guess you have to do it.

I've asked my mom, "Will I be whole when I die? When I go to heaven?" and she says yeah. She said, "You'll be just like everybody else." So I'm not scared of dying.

Another thing that got me thinking that I should take the treatments was this little guy, who, when he was five, had to have his leg amputated. He had what I had. And ever since then he's been on methotrexate, and he's still on it now. When I was in the hospital, right after I got my leg amputated, he came and showed me his leg. He was a real comfort. You couldn't tell or nothing.

When you get a prosthesis it's hard to get used to, just like anything else new. It's just like learning to ride a bike. Once you get used to it, it's very easy. You know, most people don't want to talk about it, but talking about my leg helps me. I just joke about it. My friends, when we're walking, will say, "Come on, put it in high gear." It makes you feel good to be able to joke about it. It makes it seem like it's not so bad. When other people joke about it, that brings it out in the open.

I have an easier time about the leg with kids than I do with grown-ups. I like for people to say what they're thinking. Adults pretend they're looking at a picture on the wall when they're really looking at you. But my little cousins will come up and say, "Hey, you only got one leg. Why do you have a broken leg? Why do you have to go to the hospital?"

I just don't know what to tell them somtimes. They call my leg Frank. I don't know why. And they always like to watch me dress, and put it on. I don't mind. At first they didn't understand. One day they saw me whole and the next time they saw me with only one leg. But then they accepted it, you know.

Then with football I thought, "Football is gone. There isn't anything for me to do." I had that outlook for a long time. Then I decided I was going to try to play football with one leg. There's this black guy who plays football with one leg, and he's a defensive tackle. He was in the newspaper and everything. So I decided I was going to try it. So I got on the workout program, and that's when I gained weight.

The day we were supposed to get our equipment the coach called me into his office. I sort of knew I couldn't do it, but I just wanted to *be* on the football team. And he told me, "You know, it wouldn't be good for you to do this. I'm afraid you might get out there and really hurt yourself. You haven't got enough balance to play."

I really understood his point. My brother plays football, and the coach told my brother that was one of the hardest things for him to do, to tell me that I couldn't play football. But I think he did the right thing. For football you need everything.

Sometimes I'm real depressed. I just want to get away by myself. I've often thought about just getting in the car and taking off. Just go and get my head straight. What stops me? I love my mom and dad.

You see on television all these true stories of people who are going to commit suicide, jump off a building because they're tired of living. I just wish they'd go into a hospital and look at all the little kids suffering, all the little kids that can never walk, have never walked. Kids who had surgery that didn't work.

It makes me mad that all these kids are taking LSD and smoking pot, and then kids that don't are the kids who have to suffer. I still haven't decided why me. I didn't think anything like this could ever happen to me. But it has. I think about that a lot. I asked my mom, "Why me? I mean, what have I done so bad?"

My mom told me that God picked me to suffer for other people. But sometimes I don't feel like suffering. I just want to live my own life.

Sandy Brubaker

Clipped to her refrigerator door, Sandy Brubaker keeps this poster: "I was sorry for myself because I had no shoes until I saw a man who had no feet." It's that kind of cut-and-dried philosophy she thrives on.

Sandy, nineteen, lost her arm to osteogenic sarcoma as a high school junior. She had just been voted a varsity cheerleader. So, one-armed and wearing a wig, Sandy cheered until she was black and blue and barely able to speak. Carrying a full load at school and taking chemotherapy on the side, she bore what embarrassment she felt privately.

Now a college student, Sandy majors in oral interpretation at Florida State University, not far from her home in Elkton, Florida. She hopes to use her talents as a dramatist to teach handicapped children to read.

I was a junior in high school when I got cancer. I had just made the varsity cheerleading squad when I went into the hospital for a biopsy on my wrist. A week later they amputated my left arm above the elbow.

I had just come back from Washington, D.C., on a 4-H trip. I'd carried a lot of luggage in the airport and had also been wearing a watch that was so tight it hurt. I just assumed I'd sprained my wrist. But when it continued to hurt after I got home, I went to the doctor and had it X-rayed. The doctor said it looked like an infection. So I had to wear an Ace bandage. I started out with a little elastic bandage, then got a wider Ace bandage, then this monstrosity that went all the way up my arm.

But that wasn't working at all. It really hurt. So I went in for a biopsy. I had no idea what it would be. They said it was a malignancy. I was oblivious to what in the world that meant. Cancer was the farthest thing from my mind. Even when the doctor called it osteogenic sarcoma, I assumed that was some kind of infection. Then he said, "Uh, you'll have to have your arm amputated."

The first thing I said was, "When can I get my new arm so I can cheer?" That's all I was concerned about.

That was on Monday, and the operation was Friday. The waiting was pretty routine. I had X rays. A lot of people came to see me. Some of them didn't know what was wrong, and I had to tell them. My mom said it would be harder for older people to accept it than the younger kids. That was true. It hurt my parents more than it hurt me, I think. There were a lot of kids older than I was who would come to the hospital but never come up. One guy told me later he had come but had just sat in his car and had broken down in tears.

The night they told me about the amputation, a priest friend who lives nearby came and talked. I was fine until he said it would all be different now, that I'd have to try harder. I didn't like that. From that point on I decided to make more of my life. I knew if I didn't lose my arm, I'd die. The cancer traveled from my wrist to my elbow in less than eight weeks. Osteogenic sarcoma is one of the fastest traveling bone cancers. It's a rare disease. If you've ever read the book *Sunshine*, that's what she had. She took chemotherapy in the beginning, but then she said, "Well, I'm going to live my life as a whole person." My feeling is that I'm going to live my life as a healthy person.

I tried to be completely honest with my friends. I didn't want to be pampered. I was getting help opening milk cartons and that sort of thing. My fingers weren't really coordinated.

But in that little bit of time before surgery I started trying to get used to using just one arm. You have to condition yourself if you know in advance.

The night before my amputation I just sat there looking at my fingers and thinking, "I'll never have these again." I had just gotten a manicure set, so I decided to do my fingernails. That was a very sad moment, to say the least.

I thought of it as something like getting a kidney removed. You can't stop living because of it. You're losing part of yourself, but you can't become an invalid and just stop there. If you do, you're destined for death.

I was worried about whether the other cheerleaders would feel uncomfortable having me out there with them. So when they came to visit me I took them down to the conference room and told them point blank that I really wanted to cheer, one arm or two. But I didn't want to try it if they were against it. But they said, "Of course, you're cheering. You're not stopping just because of this."

A month after the operation I went to cheerleading camp with just one arm. I learned to make the motions of clapping. It bothered me more later on, but I decided all you can do is act normal and be yourself.

I had my hair until September. My hair was nice and long—about shoulder length—but I knew it would be falling out anytime. I'd been on chemotherapy almost four months. I was sitting in school running my hand through the bottom of my hair when I looked and kind of went, "Oh, no, not now!" It was just coming out in handfuls and handfuls. So that day I tried not to brush my hair that much, but I had long strands of hair hanging down. I kept having to take off my sweater and shake it out. I went to school the next day with a scarf on and the following day I went to a beautician and was fitted for a wig. The first wig I got I hated, so I wore a scarf all the time. I cheered with that.

About eight months after my amputation I was fitted for my arm. I got it at three o'clock on a Friday afternoon, and I was cheering for a football game that night. So before the game I practiced every cheer I could think of. I practiced for three hours. It was stiff, and I couldn't swing it all the way around, but it looked so natural nobody knew I had my prosthesis on. They knew I had lost an arm, but they didn't notice it at all at first. There were a lot of stray glances, sure. I could see some people in the bleachers pointing. They were very obvious. But it didn't bother me. I figured, "Well, after I start cheering they'll say, 'Wow, she can cheer. That's cool,' and go on."

After the game everybody was going, "Oh, Sandy, your arm looks neat," and "Fantastic, let's see you move it." So I slung it up to put it in the lock position, and then I let it flop down and the joint broke! I broke it two other times. Once, I stripped the gears in the wrist from twisting it so much, and another time I broke the central bar, which is supposed to be absolutely unbreakable. I was doing a cartwheel, cheering during basketball season. Why not?

I wore the prosthesis about a year and a half. It's hard to wear it in the summer because it's so bulky. It's so hot, and it definitely shows in short sleeves.

That year I got a lot of special privileges because I had to be away from school so much. But I kept up my grades. The teachers couldn't gripe about anything. My friends, though, got really down on me because I got special treatment. I made straight A's all the way through that year.

Then I had a biopsy on one of my shoulders. I suddenly realized they thought it could come back. They were afraid a spur had gotten up into the bone marrow. I had fears then about not ever being able to marry, not living long enough to marry, and wondering if I'd have to have the bone in my stump out, and start chemotherapy all over, and that meant losing my hair. It was like getting a slap in the face. I started arguing with myself. "It can come back."

"No."

"But it *can.*"

"No."

"Yes, it can."

I was really down on life at that point. I didn't want to die. It was just one big, "Why me?" I wanted so much to be able to give the world back something good, to have a baby, a healthy baby to show the world that everything about me isn't sick.

If I hadn't gone to college I think I would have started going downhill. When I went to college I knew noboby. In class, I tried to sit up front, where you can see the board and the teachers get to know who you are. And then I went around and explained to my teachers what I had, because I knew a lot of them would wonder. I would rather have all that out of the way early in the year. It's a lot easier on me, and it's a lot easier on them. Then if another student asked it would be easier on them. Anytime, anywhere you go with an amputation, people kind of shy away. I hate to shock anybody. That's when it's hard to get in with the normal crowd at school.

Sometimes you'll be walking beside people, and they'll bump into you and they'll hit a dead end where there's not supposed to be a dead end, and they kinda look and go, "Oh."

I'm so self-conscious that if I'm at a disco place or something and a guy walks up on my good side and asks me to dance I say, "No, thank you." But if he walks up on my bad side, where the arm is missing, I'm more apt to say, "Yes."

I think not having children is the hardest for me. I was never programmed when I was younger about the possibilities of being childless. Then when I had cancer, being able to have children became even more important. I want so much to prove I'm still okay. It's still okay to be a part of me.

Emil Cohen

He was a fisherman through and through. Even when Emil Cohen became an in-patient at Tampa General Hospital in Florida, he still insisted that his mom put him into a wheelchair and roll him out to the sea wall on the hospital grounds each day so he could cast for catfish.

Leukemia forced him to drop out of high school. Yet he determined to stay in control of his life. He memorized medical lingo and became so familiar with cancer treatments that doctors special-ordered a lab coat for him. Interns new on the floor went to Emil for breaking in.

He died in 1978, just six weeks after this interview.

At the time of our conversation, Emil (say EE-mull) suffered such severe mouth sores that his mother told much of his story for him.

Emil: When my mouth sores get as bad as they are now, I eat dill pickles. It burns really bad at first, but then it numbs them. It helps. But I can't talk.

Mrs. Cohen: I don't like to see him hurt. When he's in pain, I'm in pain. Emil and I talk, and we talk a lot. I listen to what he has to say. He doesn't try to shield me from his hurt. And I cry in front of him. Sometimes when he gets into a bad disposition and gets very angry and nobody can do anything right, I'll go into the bathroom, and he'll say, "Mom, why are you crying?" And I tell him why I'm crying. I tell him, "This is not the way I'm used to seeing you. Your being sick I can handle. But this mood you're in right now I can't accept."

We've been very open about the whole thing from the very beginning. We have nothing to be ashamed of. His dad once said to Emil, "I would love to . . . if there was any way under the sun that I could take what you have and let you realize what life is all about and to grow up and to have a family."

And Emil said, "Look, Dad, if God had wanted you to have it He would have given it to you. He didn't. He chose me. This is mine. Let me handle it the way I see fit."

We can communicate among ourselves and help one another out of our depression. From the very beginning with this, we learned to accept every day as our last day, as a beautiful day. One time when I was very, very depressed, Emil told me that I was going to have to quit worrying about him, that he had leukemia for a reason. He said he was fine in the hospital. He had all the nurses and all these doctors to take care of him, and I had to get out and drive home with the idiots. And who knows, that my life might be shorter than his!

I went through a period asking, "Why my son?" at the very beginning. Our pastor came and said to me, "I can almost feel what you're feeling." He told me to know that my son is headed for a better place, it's just a matter of time . . . and Emil told us, "So I go to heaven before you. I'll just go and make heaven our home until you get there." And the pastor said, "How would you feel if they called you from some long-distance place to say your son's been shot and there's nothing you could do about it because they didn't know where he was?" I think I would feel a lot worse knowing that he needed me and that I couldn't help him.

We made his hospital room like his room at home. We decided if he has to stay here, we might as well make it more than an old drab hospital room. We have flowers and palm trees and monkeys and posters. Emil does not feel comfortable with hospital food, so whatever we're having at home we're having here in the hospital. Emil doesn't eat any of the hospital food at all.

I have a fourteen-year-old daughter who has just literally taken over at home. I felt very guilty at first, leaving them [the other children] by themselves all the time, and at first it was hard letting go. I used to go home to them every night, and Emil used to tell me I was going to have to quit worrying and fussing over him so much because he still had three sisters at home who needed me, too. He felt that even though his life could be very short, their lives had to continue and they had to grow up. They needed the same amount of care he did, he said. So I would go home, and on Saturdays and Sundays I would cook and get everything ready for the following week.

But then it got to the point where my daughter said, "Now look, you stay up here all week [at the hospital]. You need to come home and rest. Don't worry about it." She became a fantastic cook; and when Emil came home the first time, I went in the kitchen to do something and she said, "Now Mom, that doesn't go there anymore. It goes over there, because I've rearranged things to where *I* can get to them best." So I've given her the run of the house, the feeling of responsibility, and I let her know that without her Emil could not have gone through this, and neither could I. I tell her that although we've needed the hospital and we've needed the doctors, she's a bigger and more important part because she has managed and taken over and looked after her two sisters. And they also realize this, and show as much respect for Debbie as they would for me. Once, I remember the youngest one, nine, saying, "Now Mom's home. She's the mother again."

And Debbie said, "No, because Mom's resting. I'm still the mother." When Debbie tells them what to do, they do exactly that. And it makes me feel that things at home are going very responsibly. If Debbie calls on me or her dad, we stand behind her in her decisions with the girls.

I feel that when a child has any kind of illness, the whole family should be involved. Everybody should play a part. As parents, I think we should let the kids become very involved. They should be told as much as the patient knows. They should know what leukemia is, what effects it can have, and that the chances are such-and-such that it will take his life at an earlier age and that what's happening is no fun.

From the very beginning, when we first found out, we went home and told the girls. And they asked, "Well, what's leukemia?" It just seemed like immediately they wanted to find out more about it. So I said, "The best thing to do, other than my trying to explain it to you, is to just go and take a look in the medical books and the encyclopedias and anything we can find on leukemia. Let's just know what it is and everything there is to it." And we did.

We told them from the very beginning that he could die. They understood they didn't need to feel neglected, because they knew that their brother was very sick and that he needed me and that when he got better it would be their turn.

They came up to the hospital to see him, and to see the things that are happening, the things he has to go through. This helps, if for nothing else, to show them what *they* don't have to go through.

I know I've heard parents talking about children who were very rebellious, who only wanted to pick fights, who felt neglected. I'd just ask, "Do you involve them?"

And I've heard them say, "Well, they're very young."

But you'd be surprised. These kids all have minds of their own, and from what they've seen on TV they can paint this really bad picture about what all is going on—they can really become scared about what is happening—because they only know what they've seen on TV. The only way to let them know what it's like is to show them. Bring them to the hospital and let them stay part or all of a day and see, from drawing blood to starting an IV.

I feel that, as well as accepting that your child has leukemia, you go along and accept that the treatments will make him very sick. You accept that he's going to lose his hair. You accept that, chances are, it may shorten his life. It just goes on and on until you realize that little things don't matter. It's the outcome.

So I felt that losing the hair was just a little stump in the middle of the road that we could cross over by picking up our feet a little higher. We really built it up that he was going to be different, that he was going to be bald. I bought him this plaque that said, "Bald Is Beautiful" with the big kiss on the head. All his friends brought him Kojak suckers. We never said, "Poor Emil, he's gonna lose his hair." I feel the parents cause a lot of the child's reactions, because if the parent is thinking, "Somebody is staring at my child," the child will feel that.

We'd tell people, "Today he has his hair, but tomorrow it may not be there." He'd walk into church and the kids would say, "Hey, Emil, when you gonna lose your hair?"

That's the way we helped him get over the initial shock of losing it. And for a fifteen-year-old, it was hard. His hair was his pride. He had the most beautiful blond hair you ever laid eyes on. Yet I could see the excitement in Emil's face when all the nurses made a fuss over him when his hair did fall out. They'd come down and feel it, and comment about how he looked. He had a tan and was outdoors a lot, and his head tanned also. He was very muscular, and it wasn't bad looking. He'd say, "If people look, let 'em look. It could happen to them next."

Even when we went to restaurants, or to church, Emil

refused to wear a hat. And when it came back in, it was all curls. It felt like the hair on a new puppy. It had that fine, newness feel to it.

We dealt with other problems in much the same way. Emil is the kind who likes to sleep late in the mornings. So he's told his doctors that he would prefer to have his chemotherapy in the afternoon, because that way all his side-effects are over before night, before time for him to go to sleep. If he'd stay up until one or two o'clock in the morning, he could still sleep late in the morning. He liked that. And Emil would always ask for an L.O.A. [leave of absence] to leave the hospital, say, two hours, three hours before chemotherapy so he could go eat. And we would go to Morrison's or S&S, and he would just gorge himself on everything, and he'd say, "Well, I can't throw up and lose all this good food." And it worked.

Once, we were at a restaurant across the street from a funeral home, and Emil started telling me how he wanted his funeral to be: which suit, and which funeral home he wanted to go to, and that he wanted his funeral in the church, and who he wanted his pallbearers to be, the whole thing. I wanted to—as a matter of fact, I said, "We don't have to talk about that. It's a long time away." And when I got to thinking about it, well, who knows? Maybe it's not. None of us knows. Everybody's days are numbered. I feel that although Emil has leukemia, who knows, he could live to be one hundred while *I* may not take the next breath.

Medically, the doctors never kept anything from Emil. He became very involved in his blood counts. The doctors would come in and say, "Hey, what's your CBC today?" He'd call down to the lab and get his own results. And he'd say, "This is a count from how many cells?" That's when they got him his pediatrics lab coat, and they were going to let him give a seminar for new medical students; but at the time they were to come in he had no white blood cells at all. He was running real high temps, and it was cancelled.

The doctors themselves would tell the interns, "Look, if you don't know, don't hesitate to ask Emil. He can tell you." And there were a new bunch of kids starting physicals and the doctors said, "Emil, these are new students, and they have to do a routine physical. Would you lead them through it?"

And Emil says, "You start here," and he just worked them on down. That involvement made him feel in control of his own life.

Janet Lanigan

Janet, sixteen, grew up in a large, tight-knit family who promised that, come what may, they would always treat her just like anybody else. She lost her leg to osteogenic sarcoma but was back in school less than two weeks after surgery. She later got a part-time job, learned to drive, and mastered skiing on one leg.

Janet had three reoccurrences in her lungs before her death in 1978; she spent most of her last month of life preparing herself and her family for her dying.

Final remarks in this chapter were contributed by Sister Margaret Weeke, Janet's close friend.

Okay. My name is Janet Lanigan. I'm from St. Charles, Missouri, and I'm sixteen. When I was diagnosed I was fifteen. I was diagnosed with osteogenic sarcoma in March 1977.

That was when I had some pains in my knee. My right knee just swelled up and hurt really bad. Mom thought I hurt it sleigh riding. Doctors told us they assumed it was a swollen muscle, and suggested using hot towels. We did that for about a month or more before an X ray showed the cancer.

At first I thought it was just going to be a little operation. I was worried about the scar on my knee, because when you're just going into high school . . . like, you go out in a bathing suit and you think, "I don't want a scar on *my* leg." That's what I was worried about when I came into the hospital. I had no idea it would be something like losing a leg. You know?

And so I had my operation in March. I started chemotherapy, and I was on that until about the next February. Then I came back, and it was in my lung, which I was very disappointed in. Here I thought I'm on my way home, getting better. So then, let's see. I skipped a part.

I lost my hair from the first chemotherapy. That was the biggest disaster I ever faced. You'd think losing a leg would be worse than losing hair, but not to a girl.

It was a matter of life or death with my leg. What it boiled down to was do I want to lose my leg or do I have six weeks to six months to live? That's what they gave me. And so, what could I say, really?

But my hair. I thought, "No. God wouldn't. I mean, I just lost my leg. No way am I gonna lose my hair too." I thought, "Naw, I'm not being punished. It won't happen." So I just put that out of my mind and just avoided the whole idea. I made it so hard on myself, losing my hair. If I had just accepted it, I would have made it a lot easier. So that was really hard for me.

And so when it came back in my lung I was disappointed. Kinda let down. I had to have another operation on my lower lobe in my left lung. They removed that. And then I had three weeks of radiation, which I was scared to death about. I heard all kinds of rumors. You know how you pick up these ideas on TV when you're a little kid? I just got this crazy idea that it was going to turn me charcoal black. That's just the idea I picked up. And so I thought, "I don't want to be that color. I don't want to look like a piece of charcoal."

I had had no experience with it, but I was rooming with Debbie, who *had* gone through it. She could say, "It's not going to be that way." It was good that somebody who'd been through it could tell me. And then the big machines scared me. But then after the first couple treatments it wasn't bad.

Then they put me on chemotherapy, two weeks in, two weeks out, and that's what I'm doing right now. But then that's going to go on for two years.

I've had some good experiences with doctors and bad ones. In the beginning they were very open and just came right out and told me everything. They never held anything back, so I kind of got used to that because when they were telling me about having to get my leg amputated, they just came out and hit me with that. They hit me with all the chemotherapy, that I would lose my hair, and that I might not be able to have a family. I mean, one of those would be enough to handle by itself. But when they hit you with all three of them it's kind of a big blow. So I knew that they weren't holding anything back. So I had that trust that they were going to tell me everything. And my parents told me everything.

When the doctors have something to say, my mom and dad want all of us to be there. And I do, too. I think what I hear, my parents should have the right to hear. I don't think the doctors should have to explain it in two different ways. I think I'm old enough to handle it the same way they explain it to my parents. Sometimes I think I can handle it better than them. So why not just tell us together?

Before my lung surgery I was just laying there. I wasn't really scared because I'd already had one big operation—my leg. And that's a pretty major operation, from what I understand [chuckles]. And this doctor came in, and he said, "I guess you're really scared." And I wasn't until he said that! When he said that I figured, "Well, I must be scared if the doctor. . . . I guess I must be scared."

I think he was just trying to find out whether I was scared or not. I don't know.

And I think sometimes they should take into consideration the privacy. I've had a lot of problems with that. That's probably the biggest one. Like when I'm taking a bath. Okay. I don't have a leg. I don't mind being around my family. That's no problem. And around my close friends. But if I'm there and a doctor walks in, any old doctor . . . sometimes they don't think that it would bother me. I think they should take into consideration how a girl feels.

I don't know about my future. I don't even know if I'm going to be alive in the next week, so why should we sit here and try to figure it out? I think that's a waste of time. And if today's the last thing I have, then I want to make the best of that.

Because I had a threat to my life with this cancer, I've thought about dying. I'm not really scared. But it just makes me live one day at a time.

Like if I was trying to live two years from now—I have two years of chemotherapy to go—and I can't handle two years on my back right now. But if I take just two weeks at a time, that's a lot. But if I take one day at a time that's okay. I can handle it. I think it makes it easier on myself to do it like that. One day at a time. If that's the only day I have, I can make it worthwhile. It's awful hard figuring out what I'll be doing. I don't know if I'm going to have a family. Nobody living on this earth knows, really. Even if nobody ever had cancer, a threat to their lives or anything, they wouldn't know. And I'd bet you they don't think about it as much as we do, probably. I bet you they don't wonder, "Hey, am I going to be alive in a few weeks?" Maybe it would be good if they did. If everybody thought you have today, make the best of it. That's where cancer has helped me. My classmates probably never thought about dying, never thought about anything like this, and neither did I until this happened. It's been a big switch. I've changed a lot.

You know, before this happened it seemed like I had so many more friends. And for a long time I felt like I was losing them. And I just got depressed for a while, really down, thinking, "How come I'm losing all my friends?" But really I was just making a few closer ones that were going to stick by me and help me through this. But the other ones were just fake. You know how high school goes. Everybody wants to be the most popular and have lots of friends. I think those friends of mine just faded off. I just became close to a few. And I have a lot of older friends who I can talk to about more serious things. Even my closest friends in high school, one time I started talking about death to them, and they immediately turned me off. I don't know if they think I'm going to get upset and cry or something like that, or if they don't want to think about it. But I like talking to older people and to my parents sometimes. I find I can relate better. And they know I've been through this, so they treat me like I'm grown up. And so I can act that way. You know, when you're sixteen you feel like you should be treated like an adult. You think, "I'm sixteen!" But it happens little by little.

*

Janet died September 16, 1978. She kept a diary until she became too weak to write. Even then she continued to describe her feelings by telephone to her beloved friend, Sister Margaret Weeke of Cardinal Glennon Hospital for Children in St. Louis, where Janet was receiving treatment. Here is Sister Margaret's account of Janet's last days.

There's so much I could tell you about Janet and the way she died. And how well she did. She continued to worry about her family, different members of her family (they were so close), and how they were going to take hearing the news she was dying. She'd started back to school and, not knowing how long she was going to have, she put forth great effort when she went back.

But before the end of the first day, she'd gotten so tired, like by the fourth hour, that she had to call her mom and come home early.

Before she went back to school we had really talked about it. She had planned on going back full time, because she felt her mom and dad expected that of her. I told her there was no way she could handle a full day of school and that she had to compromise. I talked to her mom to see if they couldn't get her to go just half a day.

Her reasoning for going back to school wasn't that she finish school. I'm sure Janet was aware that she wouldn't live that long. I don't think she even believed that she'd live until Christmas.

One time we talked about Christmas presents, and she shared in the conversation; but when we finished, I knew that she knew she wouldn't live that long. There was no sense in worrying about Christmas presents, although she did worry about getting a family picture taken.

But when they did do the family picture she felt really bad and didn't care how she looked. But there was nothing anybody could do about that. They had the picture taken over Labor Day, which was the first chance for the entire family to be together. Some of the pictures did turn out very well.

But she went back to school a second day, and she said she just couldn't cope with her friends' reactions. They didn't know what to say to her. She couldn't smile anymore. She said she just felt too bad. And she'd have a lot of pain, and they just didn't know what to do with her. So after the second day she decided not to go back.

She had tried to tell her friends in a million different ways that she was dying, but for the most part they weren't getting the message. Especially one of her best friends. She just wouldn't believe it. I was talking to one of her friends the other night and she said how dumb she was, how long she refused to believe Janet. She said Janet would sometimes say things like, "What are you going to do when I die?" and she would just get frustrated with her for talking that way. There was a rumor going around St. Charles that she was dying, and that upset Janet because she didn't want anyone to know unless she told them herself. She was trying to tell people in due time, but she didn't want to have to handle them all at once. Janet still looked pretty well, too, which made the seriousness of her condition even harder to believe.

Her friends had a surprise birthday party for her. Her birthday was August 16. At that party she went to spend the night at this girl's house, and she was just having so much pain that when her mom picked her up that morning she was crying. Well, it scared the kids half to death. They didn't know what was going on or what was wrong with her.

Then they talked about it. They came over to her house another day and said something about this rumor going around, and she said, "Well it's not a rumor. It's really the truth." And they got all upset and said, "Oh, Lanigan, you're always talking that way." And again Janet knew that she couldn't talk to them about it.

She told one of her other friends right away that she was going to die. Although this friend wasn't sure what to do with that, she did let Janet talk a little bit about it.

Bit by bit she also talked to each one of the members of her family. She'd get upset when, for example, her mom told her sister Carol. Janet said she wanted to tell Carol herself. Later on in the evening she took Carol to her room and sat and cried for a while.

Janet prayed about how she was going to handle each situation. And one night she had been praying for Michelle. Michelle was eleven. One of the twins. And they were laying there watching a movie. Michelle was in the other bed, and Janet just felt it was the time. She really didn't feel like talking to her at that time, but she thought, "Well, maybe now's the time." And Michelle came over to her bed, and Janet said, "Do you know how bad I am?"

And Michelle said, "Yeah, Mom told me."

And Janet said, "Do you know that I'm gonna die?" And she said Michelle just started crying. She was so glad when people would cry and could let her know that they knew and that they understood. And then she could comfort them and tell them that she was okay.

For her birthday Glen, a priest, and I paid for a mini-vacation so Janet could get away. During that weekend, she had time to write six letters to members of her family.

On another night when I had spent the night at Janet's, she had talked about things you like to do before you die. I had said that I was going to write a letter saying that anybody who really knew me knew that I was happy now, and the letter could be read at my funeral.

And Janet said, "Oh, that sounds like a good idea. I want to do that."

It was scary sometimes how much she trusted me. There just seemed like there was never any doubt in her mind about whether I would lead her astray. She didn't do everything I suggested, but things that hadn't occurred to her, she just went right to them. She didn't waste time on needless things. Things that really were important, she would think about and work at.

The week before she died, her voice changed. Her neck had been swelling, and she'd been spending more time in bed. She had a whole lot more pain. And she talked about the pain. We were talking on the phone at least an hour every day. But I could tell it was getting to be more of a strain.

Her mom and dad didn't really understand why we were talking so much. I think for a while there, there were some feelings from her parents that I was taking her away from them . . . as if much of the information she was sharing with me she wasn't sharing with them.

And actually, when I work with the little children I don't let them talk to me that way. I want them to share with their parents. But I knew Janet kind of filtered the things out with me, and I could help her go back to her parents and talk to them.

She needed to do that because she was so afraid if she said this or that they would misunderstand or it would hurt their feelings or something. And I think she used me as her diary because, although she wrote in it up to the end, as long as she could, she still couldn't write in it as much as she wanted to. And by kind of spitting things out to me, she didn't need to write.

One day I called her mom, and I tried to explain that to her—that I wasn't trying to keep Janet away from her, but that Janet needed to talk about dying and that as soon as she really could talk to her mom and dad, she'd be talking to me less and less. And actually that kind of happened. It came to a point where she really could talk to her mom, and she prepared her mom. And she talked with the kids and prepared each of them. As she began doing that more and more, she talked to me less and less.

One day I said, "You know, I'm going to be coming out that way. Do you want me to stop by?"

And she said, "Well, can you spend the night?"

And I said, "No."

And she said, "Why are you going to come if you're not going to spend the night with me?"

And I said, "Well, Janet, I want to see you, but I don't want to tire you by spending the night. I know your nights are hard. Maybe over the weekend I'll spend the night with you."

And that seemed to appease her, and then she said, "Okay, will you come?"

And when I got to her house her mom carried her down the stairs into Mike's room and said, "She's really hurting. I don't know if she's going to be able to talk to you at all."

When I went in, Janet smiled, and her mom went out and closed the door. Janet said, "Now lay down. Just lay down. You just be sure you're comfortable."

And at the time I was sitting on the floor, and I said, "I want to see your face."

And she said, "Yeah, but if you're uncomfortable you be sure and lay down." So she was worried about me.

She started talking about how the kids at school were coming to visit and bringing presents. She was worried about them.

I said, "They need to do this so they feel better about themselves after you die."

Then she started talking about her dad and mom and things that were going on in the house. And she talked about her brothers and sisters, and in the midst of all that she asked me if I would ask her mom if she'd get her something to eat.

And I went out and asked her mom, and she said, "She wants something to eat?" So she got her something to eat, and she came in and sat, and we talked.

On the way out to the car then, her mom followed me, and she said, "What did you do to make Janet get rid of her pain? She said she was having so much pain when I carried her downstairs, and she hasn't eaten nearly all day, and here she sat and ate with you."

And I said that when Janet got involved in telling me about the people she really cared about and in worrying about them, she just forgot about herself. And I think that's exactly the way Janet handled things many times when she had pain. I think a lot of other kids do that, too. If you can get them involved in worrying about other people and being concerned about others, then they don't hurt as much.

On Saturday I spent the night at Janet's. Well, in the course of that evening Janet couldn't stay awake for anything. She kept apologizing. I told her she didn't need to worry about me, that as things needed to be done we could take care of them. That evening her dad, who had had a prior commitment, decided to stay home, and her sister surprised her by coming home from college, and her best friend came over. She told me that she wanted to have me sleep in the room with her. And I said okay. So I got ready for bed, and as I was going to bed I started crying, and she said, "That's okay for you to cry."

She comforted me and held my hand for a while. And then she said, "I think I'm going to die tonight."

And I said, "How come?"

And she said, "Everything's done."

Earlier in the evening I had asked her if all those letters had been written. She had had her mom write a lot of thank you notes, and they were all done, but she said she still had two more letters to do.

And I said, "Well, Janet, you could dictate them, you know. And that would be like you were writing them yourself, but your mom would be doing it."

And she said, "Well, my mom's going to have to be doing it because they're for you and Glen."

And I said, "Well, then, you don't need to worry about them."

So before she went to sleep that night she said, "Well, everything's done now."

It was a very restless night for her, a strange night. She never could share why it was strange.

I stayed awake most of the night just listening to her breathe. At one point or the other her mom gave her her medicine, and at another point Janet asked me to read to her.

I read to her from Scripture for a little while. Then she drifted off to sleep again. I could tell from her breathing that she was sleeping, but she didn't feel like she was sleeping.

That morning before I left I told her that I was going and that

I was afraid that I wouldn't get to see her again. And she asked if I thought it was going to be long, and I said it could be a day. It could be that day. But then again it could be days. She just said, "Oh, gee, I hope it's today." And I told her it would come whenever the Lord knew that everybody was ready.

Anyway, Janet told me she wasn't too good about saying goodbye and that she loved me and thanked me for sharing. She thanked me for being there when she needed me.

And it really was a goodbye. We both knew that there was nothing else to say. She was ready, and she didn't really need me anymore. It hurt very much, but it was okay.

I was away that entire week, and when I saw her again she was already getting confused. Her mother said that after that Sunday she didn't talk about dying anymore. It was as though she was finished with that. Everything was ready and in order. Her funeral was planned; the songs were planned; the singers were planned; she knew what priest she wanted, what dress she wanted to wear. She had all that taken care of. Everything was done. And then she began to get confused. She'd asked a month or so earlier if it would just get more and more painful toward the end, and I had told her that, often, kids don't need any pain medicine at all towards the end. And that's exactly what happened. She hardly needed any pain medicine the whole next week.

The swelling in her neck was very marked, and they think it was probably cutting off some of the circulation to her brain. That lack of oxygen was probably causing her confusion. But it was a delightful kind of confusion. She recognized people as they came to see her, but she was just like a little girl enjoying everything and everybody.

One of the ladies who came to see her said, "Oh, Janet, you just look so beautiful."

And Janet said, "Why, thank you. You look beautiful, too."

And just knowing Janet, she never responded favorably to a compliment. She'd always say, "Oh, how can you say that?" So it was a nice kind of confusion.

It didn't bother her that she had to be taken care of, and the swelling in her neck didn't bother her. And she could be moved with relatively no pain at all. The last three days of her life, she was awake all the time. She never went to sleep those last three days. And she just rambled on and on and on. One night I was over there, and she said, "Mom, you think I ought to have some pain medicine? Isn't it time for my pain medicine? It always makes my head feel funny."

Well, it was obvious she didn't need it. Her dad had just moved her to another bed, and it didn't bother her at all to be moved, and a week before she couldn't even tolerate being touched. And her mom said, "Well, we'd better wait until Sister leaves, or you're liable to go to sleep on her."

And Janet said, "Well, Mother, that's ignorant. You're going to make me want Sister to go just so I can get rid of the pain. Sister doesn't mind if I go to sleep on her, and besides, I'll try to stay awake."

And then we all kind of laughed, and Janet forgot about it.

She'd say, "Oh, look at those bugs on the wall. Isn't that gross? They're all lined up." And she'd laugh at them, and she'd laugh at her sister, and it kind of eased up the whole situation.

Some of the mothers (from the Candlelighters group) who were nurses were going to see her regularly, and they'd catheterize her as she needed it and take care of her other needs as they came up. Janet didn't have to go back to the clinic for the last couple of weeks of her life.

Then the day that she died, she had a spell where she stopped breathing. It scared her mom and dad to death, and they almost called the emergency squad. So then she stabilized again, and I rushed on out there.

"You know," they said, "you told us not to panic and we panicked anyhow."

And I said, "Everything in your body is going to tell you to do something when she stops. That's why you need to have somebody here with you."

I stayed there an hour, and Janet seemed stable. As I started to go, I said, "Well, Janet, let me just pray with you for a few minutes," and I prayed that Jesus would keep her at peace and that when He took her He would take her really easy. That it wouldn't scare her and it wouldn't scare her mom and dad.

And she said, "Why do you think He makes me so confused?"

And I said, "Well, Janet, does that disturb your peace?"

And she said, "No. I'm really at peace."

I said, "Well, then, it doesn't really matter too much, does it?"

And she said, "I guess not."

Then she started talking about Jello, and she was confused again. It was just a moment when she was clear as anything. That afternoon, Cheryl, a nurse who lost her daughter a few years ago, went over to Janet's at 4:00, and when she got there she realized Janet was dying.

That day Janet had seen Glen; she had seen the pastor from her church and had had confession; she had seen her best friend; she had talked to all of us, and she was in good spirits. When Cheryl told her mom and dad that Janet was dying, they and the whole family gathered around her bed as she died. Then while Cheryl did the calling, her mom could take care of the kids. They all went in and told her goodbye by themselves.

The funeral was just beautiful. All the kids in school were let out, and they made kind of an honor guard procession, and they sang the songs she wanted. I just felt so proud of her because she had done it the way she wanted to.

Martha Billings

Martha Billings grew up next door to me. Yet, by some fluke, her family moved the year Martha got cancer. That change, coupled with my own fears for her, pulled the shades down on our separate lives as though one of us had suddenly been stigmatized. It took seven years. We both finished college. Martha was married and moved to Birmingham, Alabama. We were in our mid-twenties before she and I sat down one morning over a cup of coffee and talked about what happened to her when she was a sophomore in high school. Mrs. Albert Fields, Martha's mother, contributed a parent's point of view for this section.

Martha: I was having a secretion from my breast. It didn't feel bad or anything. It was just a nuisance. I thought a lot of people had it. A nurse friend told me it was common. It was just a pain in the neck having this stuff on your bra all the time, and you know, I could feel it. The doctor gave me a pump, and I'd have to try and get this stuff out. He told me that I had a lump and that he wanted to take it out because that's what was causing me to secrete this stuff. I was glad. I was kind of chicken, but I didn't mind going in and having a biopsy.

The night before I had the operation I played football with a club at school, and I think that was the best night of my life because I almost made a touchdown. Everybody had said, "Now, don't hurt Martha," and I didn't know this. They said, "Kinda leave her alone," and I was a defensive player, and I'd go up and nobody'd be there. So a girl threw a pass, and it came right to me. And from watching football with Dad on Sundays, I knew if you caught the ball you could just run with it. So I started running, and I ran almost the whole length of the field, and everybody was hugging me. It was great.

I went into the hospital the next day, right after school. Christmas vacation had just started. The hospital was kind of fun. I'd never had my tonsils out or anything. I was just in there overnight. Then when I went to have the stitches out, we were standing in the examining room, and he told me I'd have to have another operation.

Mrs. Fields: But first, before you went home from the hospital, when he came out of the operating room, he said to me and Albert, "We're so lucky that we went ahead and did this. She's going to be just fine."

And I said, "This will be the best Christmas present we've ever had."

And as soon as Albert got to the drug store (where he works), the doctor called him up and he said, "I hate to tell you this, but your daughter has cancer. But do not tell your wife and don't tell Martha. We want them to have a happy Christmas." Albert was sort of subdued all through Christmas, but we were all so happy. He was keeping it all inside. I didn't even think there was a possibility.

Then after Christmas, while Martha was in school, her father called me and said, "Dr. Scott wants to see you in his office." He took us into his office, and he said that he was sorry. He'd sent the pathology report to three cancer centers to be sure. But the reports came back, and each one said we should go on and have the operation.

He thought fifteen was mighty young to be having a mastectomy. It was so hard to go home and face Martha. The word "cancer" to me was fatal. Especially cancer in young people. I just hated to have Martha go through it. I knew it was a very disfiguring operation, especially for someone as young as she was. I just prayed God would give Martha the strength to accept this, and He did.

So they put her back into the hospital, and they tried to do another operation without taking the whole breast. But when they sent that into the lab they found more cancer cells.

Martha: When they told me I'd have to go in for the second operation, I just thought, "Oh, damn." He told me I had a little bit of cancer, and I just said, "Well, go on and get it out." I didn't even think I'd have to go back in and have a mastectomy. It never entered my mind that it would be that bad, much less fatal. I never even thought of that. He just told me he was going to take out a wedge, and I thought, "Well, there won't be much left!" It looked all catty wampus afterwards.

Mrs. Fields: Then they told her there were more cancer cells, and they would have to do a complete mastectomy.

Martha: I think subconsciously I must have known that was coming, because I really got upset—shaking and crying—and it surprised me later on that I responded so fast. I guess going into his office with my parents was pretty traumatic. But when he said *that* I just immediately started crying. I knew something was going on *then,* but not before.

Mrs. Fields: We shed our tears behind closed doors. Martha never saw us cry. And after the mastectomy, when Martha was home, every time he'd pass her, Albert would put his hand on Martha's forehead. And I told him one time, "Martha is to lead a normal life, and she's to be treated like a normal person or she'll never make it."

After the operation Dr. Scott came out and told me, "We went under the arm, into the lymph gland, and it was clear." So I knew she would live.

Martha: Yeah, you always said that: "Everything's going to be fine."

Mrs. Fields: And then all of her friends were so understanding, and real good, especially the boys.

Martha: That was the worst part for me. Everybody knew about it. Even guys from other schools. Everybody found out about it. I was kind of embarrassed about it. I didn't want people to feel sorry for me. I thought maybe they'd think I'm real sickly. I was already skinny. But I was glad people were so nice to me.

I had had a real good year. I think that was my best year in high school. I know I was real thin and pale, and I looked sick; but I was thinking, "Well, I'm alive." I felt good. I had made it through.

I don't remember having pain, but I remember feeling real sick and groggy. But I didn't think it was that big a deal. I just knew that I was sick. I never thought I was in any danger. It was just being away from school and the fear of being treated like a freak that worried me.

When the doctor came in, oh, about three days later, or maybe a week, he took out the stitches, and I said, "I want to see it."

And he said, "Are you sure?"

I thought it would look flat, but about the same. So I looked at it, and it looked like somebody had just chewed me up, all bloodied and bruised and yellow. Oh, it looked awful. I got real upset, but at least the shock was over.

Mrs. Fields: But you know, I was waiting outside your door when he got through, and the nurse pulled the curtain around your bed because you were upset, and the nurse said, "Don't go in. I don't want you to see her upset like this. Give her time."

Martha: I think that was good, because even at fifteen, you're a person. You can figure out things for yourself. It took time for me to realize that cancer was kind of a rotten deal. Until I was a freshman in college and dating, until I started taking my clothes off in the dorm and stuff, nobody knew.

When I went out on a date, I was always afraid somebody would try something, I guess. Nothing happened. Then in college, if I dated somebody for a while I'd go ahead and tell him. One guy, I just told him that I had had a mastectomy. It took me a while to get it out. And he was surprised. He went home and told his mother, and his mother told him not to date me anymore. I just thought, "What a stupid woman." She thought I would eventually die from it or something. I thought, "Oh, that's stupid. I'm not gonna die." But it never seemed to make any difference to the guys who already knew.

Mrs. Fields: Dr. Scott was the surgeon who had done Martha's mastectomy. He felt he had done something to save her life and that was enough. But when Martha went to Dr. Butler to have her examination to go off to school, he said, "Martha, you don't have to go through life like this. I know a real good plastic surgeon in New Orleans, and I want him to see you." I said, "Let's go!" Anything that Martha wanted. It was fine with us.

Martha: I first had an operation to break up the scar, before they could implant. I was excited. I felt like the pain was worth it. I had had braces on my teeth; I had contact lenses. It just seemed like another thing to make me feel better about myself and to make me look better. I just felt like it was one more thing I had to do.

I thought it would just look perfect. I just had good hopes about it. I didn't feel like it was being vain. I think my family doctor thought that. That's one thing that kind of made me mad. He said I shouldn't have it done.

Mrs. Fields: Back then (1976) it cost us about three thousand dollars. Now, I don't know how much it would cost. We took Martha out to New Orleans just like a vacation. Made an appointment with Dr. McKee. He said in his letter that he would have to look at her before he could say. She was so flat and so thin there wasn't any skin, and that was one thing that he was afraid of. He said he'd take all that old scar off and do a zig-zag stitch and that when that heals it would make the skin stretch. He said it was fortunate that she had a small breast that they could match. They had to put her to sleep to do the first operation. It was so tedious—these tiny stitches, just like embroidery work. All the way from the middle of her breast bone to down under her arm. We were there a week. He put strips of tape all up and down, and then he had to change those. And I remember Martha had to wear her arm next to her chest while all that healed. And then in December, at Christmastime, we went back for the implant.

Martha: I felt bad about splitting the family up at Christmas. My Dad had to stay home by himself. It didn't seem like Christmas. But I wanted to have it done. I really did.

Mrs. Fields: On Christmas Eve Martha kept saying, "Let's call Daddy one more time." She said, "I just can't understand why Daddy's not home." She didn't know that Albert's boss had handed Albert an envelope that afternoon and had said, "Merry Christmas. Your plane leaves at three o'clock."

He didn't get there in time for Martha to see him that night. So the next morning, on Christmas morning, he walked in the door. Martha cried. I cried. Albert cried. The nurse cried.

And Dr. McKee said, "Put her in a wheelchair, wrap her in a blanket, and send her over to the hotel for the day." So we had Christmas Day together.

Martha: I'm sure having cancer has made me a stronger person. I might have thought my life would always be easy.

That's the only thing that's ever happened to me. I've never lost anybody I loved. I've never been sick except for that; never had any hardships. So I think it showed me that I wasn't completely lucky, that I wasn't saved from everything.

While we were in New Orleans, it was like a little vacation. We'd take a walk every night, and I remember Mom's showing me how to make a clover-leaf bracelet. It was sweet. It was a real sweet time. I felt a lot of love for Mom. I thought with the transplant, all my problems would be over. That I could wear a bathing suit, not have to wear a bra with my pajamas. It was wonderful to be able to look down and not see a big caved-in spot. I remember when he took off the bandages, and it looked good because I was laying down flat. It doesn't move, it doesn't jiggle. But when we went back to the motel I couldn't wait to take a bath. I had all this tape on me, but I could look down and see the form. And I'll tell you what, he had to put a wedge in the other breast, and I was at least a bra size bigger. It makes me rocky. It's a piece of some kind of stuff with jelly in it. They probably have something better now. He showed me what it looked like, and it was a little rubberized sack that had some fluid in it. But it's not soft.

For a long time my arm hurt. And I still don't have a lot of feeling in it, but that's the only thing that's ever bothered me. But it was just wonderful. I think anybody that has a mastectomy ought to go ahead and have it done. Just for outside looks it's fine. It's not pretty at all.

He made me, not a nipple but a pink part, and he said the last time I went back that it hadn't turned out the way it was supposed to, because it had pigmented. It has a real dark burgundy color with funny looking white and yellow things in it, spots, and it's real big and real ugly. But after what I've been through, I think this is just something to remind me that I didn't turn out perfectly.

When David, my husband, first started dating me in college, I think he just thought I was a real healthy little sophomore. But you have to tell people. They're going to find out eventually, and if whomever you tell can't take it, it's best to move on. That's a good sign that they're not worth your even caring about them. If somebody can't take something that has happened to you—something you couldn't help—then they're a weak person.

I had been dating David about three weeks before I went to New Orleans for my second operation. I thought David was great. I had never felt about anybody the way I felt about David. He was exciting. He was funny, and I could tell he knew a lot. He was really good to me. He had never tried anything. So I didn't have to tell him. But I was going into the hospital, and I thought, "Well, this is just as good a time as any to tell him."

So I told him one night that I had had a mastectomy, but that I was going to have plastic surgery and that there would be no problem. He said, "Oh." He was surprised. Later, he told me he was thinking, "Well, should I date this girl?" It didn't matter to him that I was having plastic surgery, it was just that I had had cancer.

When I came back I was really excited. I showed it to all my friends. But then, after all the bandages were off, it looked horrible. I thought it looked awful. Even so, David and I were married when we graduated from college. David is attending night law school and working during the day. We've bought a house, and in March we had a baby daughter. She's the most beautiful baby in the world!

I feel like everybody can be strong if they have to be. You have to do what you have to do. I think when you have something like this you don't think of yourself being in any other situation than the one you're in. You don't think of choices. You just adapt.

SWALLOWING IT:
THE TREATMENTS. THE TESTS.
THE SIDE EFFECTS.

. . . Why Chemotherapy?

Unfortunately, drugs used to fight cancer also damage normal cells. They can cause extremely unpleasant side effects, too: nausea, vomiting, diarrhea, and temporary hair loss, not to mention painful mouth sores.

Some people react more intensely to chemotherapy than do others. But even under the best of circumstances, doctors must limit the amount of a given anticancer drug they can administer.

Cancer cells may become resistant to the attack of a particular drug and may not be affected by it after prolonged use. Consequently, several different anticancer drugs are used at the same time or in close succession. This is called combination chemotherapy.

The vinca alkaloids, derived from the periwinkle plant, stop cell division. L-asparaginase blocks the production of the essential amino acid, l-asparagine, in certain kinds of cancer cells. Antimetabolites (say anti-mitab-O-lites) like methotrexate block the operation of the cell's normal chemical machinery. Alkylating agents such as nitrogen mustard interrupt the cell's ability to reproduce.

Patients sometimes experience a change in tastes after chemotherapy. Avoid eating greasy or overly sweet foods, rapid drinking of liquids, and over-exertion. Between meal snacks, such as milkshakes, fruit, cheese and crackers, and desserts, help put on weight. Lemonade stimulates the taste buds. Bananas, baked potatoes, meat, and milk replace the potassium lost when diarrhea occurs.

Adriamycin

This harsh, potent drug is given intravenously to avoid damaging surrounding tissue. Patients usually stay in the hospital while receiving it so that doctors can observe the body's reactions. Acute nausea and vomiting are not unusual.

The drug, a red liquid, turns the patient's urine red for a day or two after the treatment is received.

In most cases, a single intravenous injection is given once every three weeks, or on each of three days running every four weeks. A burning or stinging sensation when the drug is administered may be a warning sign that it is leaking out of the vein.

Adriamycin has been used successfully to slow down acute lymphoblastic leukemia, Wilms's tumor, neuroblastoma, soft tissue, and bone sarcoma and solid tumors.

Cytoxan

This drug is known as an alkylating agent, a chemical classification that also includes nitrogen mustard. It works against cancer cells by interfering with cell growth, much as radiation does.

It can cause immediate nausea and vomiting and can lower the production of blood cells in the bone marrow, cause hair loss, and inflame the bladder.

Cytoxan may be given either as an injection or a tablet. Drinking plenty of liquids sometimes tones down the side effects.

Cytoxan has been known to cause a change in the color and texture of the hair that grows back after treatment. (Don't be surprised if new hair comes in thick and curly and unusually soft.)

A patient's skin and fingernails may become darker during therapy. Mouth sores may also occur.

Methotrexate

Methotrexate may be taken either as a tablet or by injection. Either way, it goes to work within two hours. It has been used successfully to gain and maintain remissions, particularly in children with leukemia. It does, however, produce uncomfortable, sometimes dangerous side effects, including dizziness, headaches, blurred vision, vomiting, diarrhea, and bleeding.

After several doses, treatments may be stopped for seven to ten days to give the system a rest. Doctors may need to take frequent bone marrow aspirations during the course of treatment with methotrexate to help determine how much more the patient needs.

Prednisone

Prednisone, a drug made from cortisone, has a bitter taste but few other unpleasant characteristics. It is a white, odorless powder than can be taken in tablet form.

Those on prednisone report an increased appetite, water retention, weight gain, menstrual irregularities, and mood swings. Sometimes patients react to the drug with personality changes, insomnia, and depression. Aspirin should be avoided while receiving prednisone.

Vincristine

Vincristine is known as a mitotic inhibitor. That means it prevents mitosis, or cell division. The drug paralyzes the tumor and causes it to shrink.

Vincristine comes from a strain of the common periwinkle plant. It is used to fight Hodgkin's disease, lymphosarcoma, rhabdomyosarcoma, neuroblastoma and Wilms's tumor.

It is given by injection once a week, either directly into a vein or into the tubing of an IV. The injection only takes about a minute, but it can be extremely painful if any of the vincristine leaks into the surrounding tissue. When this happens, the injection should be stopped immediately. Any remaining drug should be given in another vein.

Among side effects, vincristine causes some people to lose the reflexes in their ankles, leaving them with a shuffling kind of walk. This side effect, as well as others, usually disappears within six weeks after the treatments are completed.

Vincristine also causes a loss of hair, muscle wasting, weight loss, and a loss of feeling in the fingers. It may also cause constipation and cramps, mouth ulcers, headache, vomiting, and diarrhea. However, side effects may be less severe in some patients than in others.

Chemotherapy in General: First Person Accounts

Jill Chapman: When I was sick, the only objective was to get well. But chemotherapy was a different story. When I was well, they were making me sick. They told me all about the side effects, but at the time it went in one ear and out the other.

Robert Needham: Just keep thinking, "If I go through this now, I'll feel better later." It's a help.

Janet Lanigan: We called them my green-bucket days.

Wayne Pelron: The medicine makes you sick so fast you won't have time to run out the door. You just have to throw up. But after a while everybody gets used to that. You learn to recognize the symptoms.

Anonymous: Once you get off the medicine, it's hard to lose weight. It's like learning how to eat all over again. When you're on chemotherapy, you don't have to worry about it. When you're sick, people keep telling you, "Oh, it's so wonderful you're gaining weight. Gain some more." Now I don't have all the medicine, and it really shows.

Cheryl Hall: Before I started on vincristine my face was really breaking out. But I tell you, my face has never been so clear. I can't believe it.

Sandy Brubaker: After I got off chemotherapy, zit, zit, zit, zit,

zit. As soon as I got off it I didn't have the medicine cleaning my skin out.

Dana Ensley: I think you should do everything you can to prolong your life and enjoy it while you can, even if it means taking chemotherapy. Just ask yourself, "Would I rather die than take chemotherapy?"

Tim Sperandio: Adriamycin changed me. I was in my own world. Seemed the minute it was in my veins, I'd turn into a monster. One point I was all nice and the other point—when they put me on the drug—I was crabby. I was always sick and getting diarrhea from it.

I felt I was being punished for something, and I didn't know why. I got these feelings like I'd lived before and I might have been like Adolph Hitler. I used to go up to my room and sit there and wonder, "What have I done to have this happen to me?"

Brenda Washington: Adriamycin is that red stuff they put in your veins. It burns like mad. But if it's going to keep you alive, you take it. You don't fight it.

Valerie Nelcamp: It got to the point where anything I saw that was red, be it Jello or a cherry soda or anything that I came near, I would get sick, just seeing it. Even though it's all in your head, it's a real sickness.

Eddy Kimball: When I first started into chemotherapy treatments, I was taking cytoxan, which really makes you deathly sick, you might say. I would get it on Friday morning, and I would be sick until Sunday afternoon, nonstop. Vomiting. It was pretty bad. I would get dehydrated sometimes. It was just no fun at all. I had no weekend at all, and school was all of the rest of the time. Eventually I started getting sick and nauseated before I would ever get the medicine. When I walked in the door of the clinic, I'd get sick. And when they started the IV, I would start up right then, because it tasted awful. You can taste it when you get it IV.

Well, a psychologist, Dr. Cooper, suggested hypnosis and taught me how to do it. It worked most of the time at the very first, and then I guess eventually it was myself who stopped the throwing up so much. I would throw up maybe once when I got the medicine and once when I got home. And the next morning if I woke up and would eat right away I would have a decent weekend.

Tracy Klinko: When you go to the hospital you can smell the treatments. And you can't drink anything when you're supposed to. The only thing that makes me sick is cytoxan and vincristine together. You can set the clock by it—you throw up violently for ten hours, and in ten hours to the minute it stops.

Alane Morehouse: Prednisone makes you real puffy in the face and makes your stomach bulge. It gives you a real good appetite. You just eat and eat and eat and eat. The pills are very bitter, so you've got to swallow them real quick or they'll drag down your throat. I had to take four a day when I first started—to control my fever. I hated it. I used to flush them down the toilet. But it didn't make any difference. It didn't make my appetite go away, and it didn't make my face get any skinnier. I had cravings for things like artichokes—we had to have them every night. I remember hiding the pills under the edges of my plate at the table.

Millie Thomas: With prednisone they told me to expect a ravenous appetite, and that I might get hooked on something like bread or spaghetti. I decided if I was going to get hooked on something it was going to be on lettuce with dressing that had two calories per tablespoon. Which I did! So I didn't get fat. But with prednisone, hunger is a physical pain in the middle of your stomach. If you can wait for about fifteen minutes, the feeling will subside. Then go and get a green salad, and it'll be okay.

Lisa Robison: On prednisone I'd just about eat another supper before I went to bed. I'd get up at three in the morning and eat.

Jill Chapman: On prednisone I got a taste for Cheez-its and that made problems with my complexion. I got real live zits because I was always eating these Cheez-its.

Home Remedies for Green Bucket Days

Dehydration—Eat jello. Suck on ice. Make and eat ice cubes made from fruit juices.

Nausea after eating—Eat smaller meals more often.

Weight gain caused by prednisone—Keep away from starches. Eat fresh fruit. Cut down on salt.

Weight loss—Drink protein-rich milk shakes (mixed with egg). Eat rare steak, cheese, nuts. Drink eggnog.

Vomiting—Sleep after chemotherapy. Drink flat ginger ale. Eat hard boiled eggs. Have a light breakfast before going for treatment. Avoid milk.

Diarrhea—Eat rice, cheese, eggs, potatoes, and bananas.

Constipation—Drink prune juice. Eat natural cereals, fresh fruits, and vegetables.

Continuous nausea—Eat mints.

Radiation

Radiation stops the cell from dividing and eventually kills it. Because cancer cells grow faster than normal cells do, they are more vulnerable to the radiation.

Radiation can be used to shrink a large tumor to a size a surgeon can remove, or to knock out cancer cells before they become dangerous to the patient. It can also relieve bone pain.

Radiation does not reach deep-lying organs and rarely causes permanent side effects. There may be a feeling of fatigue after radiation, and a redness of the skin where the radiation was aimed. Some patients say they have trouble swallowing afterwards. The skin may itch and peel, which can be helped by applying corn starch.

Tim Sperandio: For two solid weeks after the radiation, I couldn't put an ounce of solid food down. It was malts, malts, malts. It felt like my throat was closed together. When we had Thanksgiving dinner Mom made everything, and I sat down and took one bite and started crying. I was so hungry, but I couldn't eat it.

Anonymous: You can smell it before you even go into the radiation room. You get so sick and nauseous. I'd walk into that X-ray room, and I remember smelling that shampoo, and to this day it makes me sick to smell it. But while I was taking it, I'd think to myself, "I'd rather get sick now than die later." I mean, *really*.

Bone Marrow, Blood Tests, and Spinal Taps

A *bone marrow biopsy* and aspiration, or bone marrow for short, helps doctors tell if the body is producing healthy blood cells.

To do the biopsy, a needle must be inserted into one of the bones. It can be painful at first, and may leave a small bruise afterwards. But the test only takes about five minutes, and the area can be numbed first.

Sometimes the patient lies face down on an examining table, and the needle is pushed into the back of the hip bone. When the needle is withdrawn, it contains the thick, red bone marrow that goes to the lab for examination under a microscope.

When the test is over, most people feel well enough to get up and go on about the day's business; some patients say that standing up too soon after the bone marrow causes a headache.

A *blood count* shows how many and what condition the white and red blood cells are in. A healthy blood count averages five thousand to ten thousand leukocytes and two hundred thousand to three hundred thousand platelets responsible for clotting.

To make the blood count, a laboratory technician examines a sample of blood under a microscope. A ruled area is used to divide the cells into small squares. Sometimes the blood is stained to help distinguish the characteristics of the red blood cells and the variety of the white ones. Some blood diseases and inflammations can be recognized in this way.

The examiner also looks for the percentage of hemoglobin in the blood, how long the blood takes to clot, and whether it contains parasites.

The test takes about five minutes. Sometimes blood can be obtained by simply pricking the finger. Sometimes a syringe is used to withdraw larger samples from a strong vein.

A *spinal tap* is performed by inserting a needle into the spinal cord in the lower part of the back. By extracting fluid from inside the spinal column, the doctor can tell if cancer cells have begun traveling toward the brain. By injecting medicine directly into the spinal column, this spread can often be prevented or avoided.

To make the test, the patient is told to lie on his side. The needle goes between the second and fifth lumbar vertebrae. A headache afterwards is not unusual.

Wayne Pelron: They tell you to get down over your knees and hold your breath [for a bone marrow]. But you're shaking so bad that you can actually feel the weight of the needle bouncing on your back. One thing I found that helps a lot is to crack a joke. I always say, "Little stick, my foot! You guys lie enough to be politicians."

Robert Needham: If you relax, it won't hurt so much. Just think about something else, something really good that happened to you, and forget about what's going on behind you.

Tim Sperandio: Your brain's floating in a jelly, the way I see it, and when they start taking that out, with a spinal tap, it lowers your brain. If you stand up straight right away after they get done with you, you'll wind up with a headache like anything. Lay there for a little while, then get up.

Robert Needham: They used to come in every day for blood tests, and I'd get really miserable and move my arm around and try to make them not do it. But when I realized that was one of the things that had to be done, I calmed down a lot. Just think about getting it over with so they can find out what's the matter and give you the medicine to help.

Amputation/Fitting a Prosthesis

Janet Lanigan: What it boiled down to was, "Do I want to lose my leg or do I have six weeks or six months to live?" That's what they gave me. And so what could I say, really? Another girl who had had the same thing came and talked to me and showed me her false leg and how it worked. So I was all prepared for what I was about to have. That really helped a lot. Seeing that someone else had gone through it and how happy she was, and how her leg really didn't matter, helped.

Anonymous: I had never heard about prostheses or artificial legs. I thought I would be in a wheelchair. Then the doctor told me you could do almost anything. The night before my surgery, another kid who was going to have the same thing came in and talked to me about it. In talking to him, I got over my fears, and that was really helpful. I made up my mind to do a lot of things. I thought about it every day. Then when I got my prosthesis I learned how to walk and act, and I have done real well since. I play basketball and baseball, and lately I play a lot of golf. One of my coaches at school asked me to kick field goals this year in football, so I've been practicing a lot. I'm going to try really hard to do that.

Renee Brown: It didn't take me five minutes to decide when they told me the alternatives to amputating. I just said, "Go ahead." I would have had no use of my leg. It would have been without all the muscles and nerves.

My parents knew because the doctor told them, but I made

the decision. I didn't want a paralyzed leg. I wanted to be able to walk. I wanted a chance to get on with my life. Otherwise it would have spread too fast. I just thought about that. But about a month afterwards, it really hits you. You feel pretty bad, and if anybody says anything to you about it you get really upset. It's like any major operation. You get down for a while and then you're fine.

I got my leg about two months after the operation. My stump healed really fast. The prosthesis was a suction kind, with a hole in it where you put the stump, then screw this thing in to squeeze all the air out. It has no straps or anything. I could walk really good with that. But every time you lost or gained a pound, it affected the way it fit and the way you walked. So I went back and got another one which has a strap around the waist, and although I don't walk as well with it, I wear it more. Cosmetically, it looks real and feels real. About eight months after my amputation, I walked thirteen miles in a cancer walk-a-thon. You have to prove yourself—not to others, so much, but to yourself.

When somebody says to me, "Oh, you can't do that," it's my nature to want to do that very thing. I'm so stubborn. I've learned to dive balancing on one foot, and I think I could probably ski that way. I balance on one foot all the time. I don't think about the negative aspects much. If you're on a baseball team, you don't sit on the bench and say, "Oh, we're going to lose."

Steve Bennett: Before I had my leg amputated, I'd see people with one leg and I'd stare. Now when I'm in a mall and I see people staring, I understand. You can't help but stare when you see something different. But I don't like somebody to pretend they're looking at a picture on the wall or something when they're really glancing at my false leg.

I had a cane, and I named it Elmo from a cartoon I was

watching on TV one morning. I just started calling it Elmo, and then all my friends started calling it Elmo. It just got to be a fun thing.

Sandy Brubaker: When I explain it to young children, I say I had cancer in the bone, and it was traveling up my arm. I tell them that if I hadn't had my arm cut off I might have died. That translates something bad into something good, something they can understand. I often tell little kids that some day I'm going to be like the bionic woman, that maybe I'll get a new arm sewn on just like she has. Sometimes I believe that. Then when I show kids how I tie my shoes one-handed, they say, "Oh, terrific! Lemme try it." If I can get them to touch my stump, it's even better. I pretend I'm a waiter and drape a towel over the stump, or paint a little face on it, put a wig over it, give it a name, put a plastic glove on it and blow it up, make it talk . . . anything to get the kids to laugh, to help them relax, to get over their fears about it. During the summer, I rarely wear the prosthesis because it's so bulky and hot.

But when I *do* wear it, you'd never guess it's fake. It was cosmetically matched to my arm. They first took measurements of my joints, fingers, arm length, everything. Then they took pictures (of my good arm) and matched skin color. They made a plaster mold of my stump, then built an arm that fit over it. The prosthesis cost about fifteen hundred dollars. The Cancer Society helped pay for it. When you pay that much for something you can't just throw it by the wayside.

Valerie Nelcamp: I knew that I would have to have surgery, but I didn't have time to suffer and agonize over it. They told me that osteosarcoma was a life-threatening disease and that without the surgery my chances were dangerously slim. I knew then that I would have to do this in order to gain my life, that it was the price I would have to pay for my life.

THE HOSPITAL SCENE: TAKE A WALK IN THE ZOO

On the Inside: Nurses, Night Stalkers, and Other Goofs

Malcolm Schorlemer: Sometimes it seems like the nurses refrigerate their hands.

Jill Chapman: I really don't like it when the interns stand outside the door talking. They don't stand outside my door and talk about me, but they stand there talking about somebody, and I know that at one of those doors they're talking about me.

Anonymous: This new nurse came on the floor one night. I wanted to kind of break her in. So I poured apple cider in the urinal, and when she came in to take it, I pulled it out from under the sheets and held it up to the light. Then I said, "Gee, looks kinda cloudy. Better send it through the filter again," and drank it. That wiped her out.

Alice Demick: In the hospital they really take away your personality. They take away your clothes, your privacy, they decide your schedule, when you take a bath, when you eat. All the bars are down. And if they don't explain anything, it can be really traumatic. You feel like an object that's out of order the doctors are trying to figure out.

Debra Vehlewald: I know Cardinal Glennon is a learning hospital, but I don't like all those people coming in and gawking at me. I've had a couple of doctors who, just because they were specialists for chest tubes, have come in and done stuff. That upsets me. They don't know *me*. They don't understand me. I can't talk to them at all. If they'd just tell me what they're going to do, you know, I'd work with them. It's no big deal. But they come in and start doing stuff, and I'll ask them what they're doing and they'll say, "Well, we're just going to do this." If they'd say, "I'm going to free your tube, or re-arrange it, or tape it, take it out . . ." whatever, I'd work with them. They just never did.

Jill Chapman: I was older than a lot of the kids in the hospital, and they always said, "We like you because you don't kick and fight when we stick you." I didn't kick, but I did fight. I fought with words! So I felt like they appreciated the fact that I *was* older. I've always been stubborn anyway. I appreciated having an equal chance to say something. Dr. O'Connor can tell you that they [the doctors] can't just sit down and say something. I cross-examine them. But if they know something they don't think I should know, they should at least give me a satisfactory answer. I don't think they should tell me something if they aren't sure, because that doesn't do me any good. I have enough worries of my own.

Tim Sperandio: There were times when they've asked me how I felt and I felt miserable, but I said I felt good because I was afraid they'd do something more to me.

Emil Cohen: When they come in late with the treatments, that's when I get sick, and I tell them, "The reason I got sick is because I've been sitting here waiting for you all to come in. I have to sit here and wonder if the next person that walks in is going to have something for me." You just tell them. That's the only thing you *can* do.

Jeremy Varick: Always when I go into the hospital, even when I'm not getting anything, I feel down and not as good as I did before. But after a while I perk back up. When you know you're getting something (chemotherapy), most of the agony is worry—worry about the pain, the bone marrows, and spinal taps. If you get sick before you get it, that's from worrying. I worry all the time. I really kind of have to.

Millie Thomas: I had watched *General Hospital* on TV, and in those shows everybody that goes into the hospital falls in love with the doctor. But it's not like that. And if you go in there expecting it, you're going to unconsciously set yourself up for this situation. When you're in the hospital flat on your back, all alone, it's very easy to fantasize about crushes and romance.

Emil Cohen: At the first, my doctor said she could either tell me what's coming at the last minute or a week before or the day she decides on it. And I said, "When you decide, I'd like a week's notice." You just get used to it. If you're going to get stuck, you're going to get stuck. There's no way of getting around it. You might be able to put it off for a day or so, but that's about it.

Some people prepare themselves to get sick. A lot of times I'll say, "Scratch my arm, Mom, do something different, scratch my head," and I'll say to myself, "I'm not going to get sick, I'm not gonna get sick," and sort of psych myself up to how good it feels that she's scratching my head or something like that. It drives me away from the feeling of nausea. Then it passes.

Face to Face With Doctors

Jill Chapman: I think when the doctor tells the kid face to face instead of telling the parents, it helps the parents realize that it's the kid's problem. I always resented it when my doctors asked my parents to step out in the hall with them to talk about my case.

Kenny Marsh: The doctor should tell the patient straight out what he's going to have to go through, unless the patient doesn't want to know. You're the one making the decisions.

Lisa Robison: The doctor won't tell me anything. He'll tell Mother, but he won't tell me. And I'm sixteen.

I think I'm adult enough to hear it. I want to hear everything. If he said, "You've got two weeks to live," that would be fine and well. I could get out and do things I really want to do. But if he waits until I've got two days and tells me, I mean, what am I going to do with two days? He doesn't want me to get all upset. But he doesn't want me to think I'm going to be cured, either.

Tim Sperandio: I think the meanest thing a doctor could do is not tell a patient. The doctors never told me what the consequences of leukemia are. They only told my mother. When I took myself off chemotherapy, my mom told me the consequences. I was shocked. She said I had five years to live. When I found that out, I was mad at the doctors; because the way I see it, it's my life and they should tell me. I should be ready for death. I'm not scared of it. It's even harder on the parents who wait until five years later, when you start getting sicker and sicker, and you're laying there in the hospital dying, and wondering why. I think anybody over thirteen can accept the fact and should know.

Anonymous: The doctors used to tell me, "Never give up hope." I got sick of it. And it made me wonder if there was a reason I didn't know about that would make me give up hope. It kind of throws you off the track when they say that.

Jill Chapman: They told me all the things that would happen so fast that, later, I couldn't remember whether they said if I could have brain damage or not. I thought, "I don't know about that. Did he say that?" To this day I haven't asked the doctor if I can have kids. When I wanted to ask, my mother was always there, and I'd hate to admit in front of my mother that I was thinking about this problem. I didn't want her to know if I couldn't.

Debra Vehlewald: They just don't say anything unless you ask. Not to me, anyway. I was scared to ask. I didn't know what was going on, and I felt that if they wanted me to know they'd tell me. If my mom's there, she'll ask this and this; she'll say, "She doesn't need to know that right now, spare her from this, and tell her this part." It's upsetting. But when it's just me there, I can ask these doctors what's going on and what I'm going to go through.

Alice Demick: When a doctor makes you feel like he's in no hurry, and sits on the bed and asks you what you want to talk about, you really feel like that doctor cares about you.

It's really aggravating when you go to a doctor, and he doesn't remember your history, doesn't remember your case, when you've been to him ten times. You think, "How can they know what to do? If they have that many patients. . . ."

Jill Chapman: While I was on nitrogen mustard, one doctor became very special to me. He'd come in and say, "What do you want? Mustard, relish, or catsup?" With him I knew he respected me as a person. He let me talk. He gave me a chance. I like a doctor who doesn't treat me like I don't know myself. Simply because he made me feel like I was important as a person made it all worthwhile for me.

Anonymous: When the doctors suggested I talk to other kids, patients with cancer, that really started my mouth moving. Getting to know them and answering their questions made me feel good about it. Afterwards, I could hit it off with anybody. I really opened up.

Jeremy Varick: The bad thing is, when you have a relapse they always tell your parents first. They shouldn't do that. They should tell the kids first.

When a Cancer Friend Dies

Anonymous: I used to get really shook up when somebody in the hospital I knew died. I used to think, "What if it's me next?" Then I would say to myself, "No, it's not going to be." You have to say that.

Alane Morehouse: One little boy in the hospital with me had leukemia. One week I saw him running down the hall swinging his IV bottle, and the next week when I went in they said he had died.

I said, "But how? I just saw him."

That scared me. I thought, "If it could happen to him . . ." They said he had tumors behind his eyes. That scares me because when I get headaches around my eyes it makes me think, "Oh, no. Am I getting tumors behind my eyes?" Sometimes my eyes burn bad.

Dana Ensley: When you lose a friend, it takes a long time to get over it. But you have to look at it this way: Every person's case is not the same. And just because this person died doesn't mean that you will.

Jill Chapman: When Janet [Lanigan] told me they had tried all these drugs that didn't work for her and that they didn't have anything left to do, that scared me.

I thought, "Doesn't sound very good to me."

I was numb. I didn't cry. Maybe I didn't believe it. There

was nothing I could do, and by getting upset I couldn't help her, so I just sat around and wondered.

I really respected her for telling me, because she knew what I was thinking. She knew I would understand what she was really saying. I had the same hope that she did that she would never get sick again, and that she'd be okay. That she wouldn't have to worry about it for a while, anyway.

But then she told Sister Margaret, "If Jill comes home from school and I'm dead, she's going to be so mad at me," then I knew she must realize it.

I know when I joke about something, either I'm testing somebody to see how they react or I'm testing myself to see how it sounds to say it. She knew good and well. She was just getting ready.

Sandy Brubaker: I knew one girl who went through so much: three amputations on her leg and tumors in both lungs. *But* she just kept taking it. She never complained, she never said, "I hurt, I need an IV, help me with something." She did it on her own. She was very much an inspiration.

Alane Morehouse: All you can think of that comforts you is that the person is out of pain.

Tracy Klinko: My parents have some friends whose little boy died of leukemia when he was two. So last summer I spent two weeks with them, and it reminded them a lot of their kid. It made me really happy.

Traumas Over Medical Bills

Jill Chapman: We were a regular, middle class family. I never had to worry about money. But when I got sick it worried me because the hospital expense was so bad. Somehow I found out what it cost per day, how much it was going to cost total, and it really bothered me. And I told my dad one afternoon, and he said that he was kind of worried about it, too, but that he had just gotten a job to build an apartment complex and that the money from that job would take care of it right there. And I felt so relieved when he told me that. It seems like every time something hurts there's something to make up for it. Once my dad said to me, "You know, your insurance payments are really important. When you get married, make sure you pay your insurance before you eat." I know it was a real burden. But my father already knows I'm going to be an expensive child to raise. He said to my boy friend once as we were leaving, "You know she's expensive, don't you?"

Millie Thomas: My parents always assured me that no matter what happened, money was no object. They were afraid I would be tempted to say, "Hey, let's stop this treatment. It's costing my parents too much money." I think if I ever *did* stop the treatments because of money they would be severely disappointed in me because I didn't think I was worth the price. They always made me feel that I was worth everything to them.

Robert Needham: When your parents pay so much, that's

their way of showing how much they love you, how much they care for you, and how much they want you there.

Alice Demick: The bone marrow transplant was extremely expensive. There was no way we could afford it. I don't have a father. My father left us when I was six weeks old. I'm the youngest of nine children. So when I had the bone marrow transplant, there was a fund raised. My high school English teacher raised close to fifty thousand dollars. She got an article into the newspaper, which I was not crazy about. I did not like being publicized. But charity is a good thing for all people to experience. In my case, people had marathons, and they had a benefit dance and bingo games and raffles. She (the teacher) just set at it and did it. Everybody's charitable. Maybe not always with money, but with thoughts and ideas, helping, volunteering. If you have a hard time accepting charity, take it anyway and give something back. Say thank you. That's a big thing. It's really all you can do. You can't feel indebted all your life.

Tim Sperandio (Tim's mother, unemployed and a former cancer patient herself, contributed to this segment): Frankly, we're very poor. My mom is raising two teenagers alone. When we lived in Denver, Medicaid picked up everything. It wasn't until we arrived in Missouri that we found out we couldn't get it here. Even the United Fund told me to go back to Colorado. They wouldn't help us.

We had a bad scene when we came to the hospital, and they said, "You know, we're not a free hospital." Both of us were crying. Finally they said that it was okay, that we could charge it. Now we have huge hospital bills facing us. We kept getting calls from the Lions Club saying they wanted to run an article to help raise money, but the reporter called about six weeks ago and we haven't seen the story yet. They're always *going* to do this and *going* to do that, and then we don't hear from anyone. I don't plan ahead anymore because it just ends in letdowns.

Karen Jepsen: If your doctor will declare you disabled, you can qualify for disability under Social Security, possibly under your parents. You have to have worked for a required number of quarters. Once you're declared disabled, you can qualify for vocational rehabilitation. Through this, I'm getting some money for college this year.

HEARTBREAKS
AND
HANG-UPS:
FACING THE WORLD

Going Bald

Frances Grimes: The day before I went into surgery a nurse came in and sat down and told me that I would lose a great deal, if not all, of my hair. I had long blond hair.

About two months after I started the chemo, I lost all of it. One night I was brushing my hair, and it started falling out all over the bed. My cousin came in, and he was brushing it; but he didn't know it was falling out, and a big bunch of it came out on the brush. He didn't know it was supposed to do that, and it upset him so much he said he could have gone out on the doorstep and cried for years. And I was upset for him to see that. I didn't look in the mirror for a week. Then I went into the shower one night, and I saw it. Momma said, "Well, it's the good Lord's work. He's taking care of you and so is the doctor."

I would sit there and rub Vaseline on it. They said if you would do that your hair would come back in. I'd go outside about two hours every day and let the sun hit me. It took about six months to grow enough hair to go without a scarf. It came in straight the first time, but the second time it curled and I had a cowlick in the back. It came in brown. You could look at a picture of me then and the way I am now, and you'd say, "That's not her, is it? That *can't* be her."

Anonymous: My mom keeps asking me if I want a wig, but I say, "No." I'd rather have my hat pulled off than a wig. It'd be more embarrassing if I was wearing a wig.

Cheryl Hall: Once my sister and I were sitting on the curb at the movies, waiting for my mom, when this gang of girls came up to us and started kidding me about my wig. I could see they wanted trouble, so I yanked off my wig and said, "You touch me and you'll catch it, too." They turned around and got out of there!

Jeremy Varick: I'd wear these mesh hats that other people could see through. But I'd rather for them to see through it than for me to wear a solid hat and them not be able to see. I kind of want everybody to know.

Wayne Pelron: When you lose your hair, it's not like you're going to die. You won't stay bald forever.

Columbus McRae: One night I was sitting while my sister platted my hair, and a big ole plat of hair came out. I was scared. I didn't know what was wrong. My doctor hadn't even told me, so I didn't know. It just kept on falling out. When I went back, I asked my doctor why he hadn't told me about it so I wouldn't have been scared by it. He told me next time he would.

A heap of people asked me what happened to my hair. I told them. Talking takes a lot off my chest. I started wearing a hat some, but it was too hot. I stopped wearing it. I didn't feel embarrassed, or when I did, I told myself it was better than being sick.

Alice Demick: We are a very hair-conscious society, so people who lose their hair *do* feel very uncomfortable, especially in a group. People give you weird looks.

Emil Cohen: I feel that I'm the same person without hair as I was with hair. There's no difference. You're still the same person. Why should it bother you? Don't worry about it. If people look at you, let them look. Who cares? You're the same person no matter *what* happens to you.

Anonymous: My hair fell out about two weeks after chemotherapy. It was real thin anyway, so it didn't really take much to fall out. But my parents didn't let me have the mirror, and when I finally got them to, it was not really that bad. It was just the first shock of it.

I went around with friends in my neighborhood without my wig. A lot of my friends knew about it, and friends told friends and everybody knew. It didn't bother me. It didn't bother them, either. Or if it did they didn't let me know.

Dana Ensley: For a while there, losing my hair really got to me. Nobody wants to lose his hair. But then I got to thinking that there are so many people who lose an arm or a leg or maybe even their eyesight. Your hair can always come back. Eyesight can't. That's the way I looked at it, and I was able to say, "Okay. I'm thankful I've got my arms and my legs. And I don't have to lose *them.*"

Jeremy Varick: When I first got chemotherapy, my hair did not fall out. I wasn't expecting it to, either, because I didn't know it was supposed to. So when I had my relapse the first time, I kept thinking, "If my hair didn't fall out last time, it won't fall out this time." So when it did, it was a shock. I've learned that when you lose your hair, wearing a hat actually slows the growth of your hair down. This last time, it came out, but not all of it. I still had some long hair. In some people it comes out in spots. In mine, the back didn't come out. In fact, I had a line of hair around my head, and it looked stringy and dumb. It's worse when you're like that. So my dad got the idea to just go ahead and cut it off. He was right. It helps when it grows back because it'll all grow back evenly.

I was bald half a year in sixth grade, and then in seventh. At the beginning of the year my mom went in and told all of my teachers what my problem was. So I had permission to wear the hat. But when it's embarrassing is when the teacher tells everybody else to take their hats off and everybody's yelling at you, "Take your hat off."

You just say, "No, I've got permission." What would really be good, and I'd wish they'd do, I wish before I went in they'd just tell all the kids that I was going to be in class with them. You end up telling them yourself. Somebody always gets curious and says, "Why does that kid wear a hat every day?"

Tracy Klinko: I've got a toupe. Nobody knows I've got it except my mom and dad and brother. A toupe is a man's wig.

When I had my hair and it began falling out, it was only two weeks before school started. So we bought a toupe. It's got a little tape thing on it that keeps it on your head. It makes me feel more secure. When I didn't have it, the kids would laugh at me. And the only way you could get them not to was to go through this hour-long talk telling them what you've been through. So we decided instead of wasting twenty hours we'd spend twenty dollars.

Karen Jepsen: I hated being bald; I hated wearing my wig. I hated talking to anyone about it. I wore my wig, outwardly pretending it was my hair, but hating it. I only let a few select people see me without my wig on. A year later I quit college after one quarter because my hair had started falling out again, and—afraid it would all go—I chose to quit rather than to wear a wig. A year later, when I lost my hair for the second time, I could accept what the doctors had always said before: Being bald and able to take medicine is better than having hair and being dead. Yet it's taken me three years to come to this acceptance. Doctors, nurses, people in general have to understand the psychological strain it can cause.

How Parents Cope

Jill Chapman: Most parents have a real hang-up about their kids. When I became a teenager, I was still kind of babyfied. When you get on up fourteen, fifteen, sixteen, what you've succeeded in doing is getting yourself right smack in the middle of nowhere. You're not a kid, and you're not an adult. There's a lot of things you don't know yet. Thousands of basic things. You're just naive.

Your viewpoint is from an in-between place. And your parents are looking at you and worrying like crazy and hoping that you don't stay like that forever. They want you to go on, but at the same time they realize that you just came from being a child. They're kind of stuck. So they have to use a trial and error approach to see what's going to work. Probably what their parents used for them. That's the only way to learn: to ask questions, to guess, to try.

As I got older, my parents would often tell me they thought I was more mature than my friends. Then they'd turn around and get mad at me and take my allowance away, or something really dumb like that. Here I was, supposed to be so mature, and so responsible, and they were treating me like a child. They had to protect me, out of love. They didn't want me to get any sicker, and they felt that was what they had to do.

Anonymous: The best thing your parents can do is to treat you like the same person you've always been.

Millie Thomas: I know I must have put my parents through hell, just because they had to deal with me every day, and I was completely unaware that I had cancer. They had to go around acting like everything was okay. It must have torn them apart.

Tracy Klinko: The most you can do for your parents is to do whatever they tell you to do. Act like you're not scared, even if you are. Do a little more than what they ask you to do. Make them feel proud. Most parents who have kids like this know what's going on before the kids do.

Anonymous: My father feels real guilty. He never had time for us. Even now he's got to think about his crops. He doesn't have time to sit around and pat the top of my hand.

He never asks me to do anything because he always thinks I'm so tired. It would help if he would just go back to the normal way of treating me. I mean, I wouldn't mind if we had fights every day. Now it's gotten to where anything I want I get. He doesn't want to do anything to alienate me.

When I was in the hospital, I was sick. That was fine, to get anything I wanted. But now, I can just mention it, and it's there. Like my new car. My daddy said, "You want that car?" I said, "Yeah, if you want to buy it." And he came up the driveway and said, "Here's your birthday present."

That's it. It's guilt. I think it's really sweet that he's so considerate, but I hate him feeling I'm going to die all the time. Daddy doesn't expect me to, but he knows I'm going to do it one of these days. It worries him. He's paranoid.

Mother is a worrier. She worries too much. When I get sick, she's sick. The doctors tell *her* what medicines I should be taking. She asks him to repeat it over twice, sometimes, and that embarrasses me. I can catch it. I feel like they should tell me that stuff alone.

And then she says, "We are going to be taking this," and "We are going to be taking that," like both of us had to take it.

Nobody else can understand. When Mother gets on my case, I just don't feel well; I don't want to talk to her; I feel like crying.

I hate to be stared at, especially when I'm trying to sleep. Sometimes she gets so nervous it makes me nervous. But I can't say anything, or she'll feel hurt.

I think if your family pretends you're going to get well, they're only fooling themselves. And when they sit around and cry, that can *really* get to you.

Steve Bennett: It's good when your parents cry openly. It shows they're hurting just like you are. And they love you. I've only seen my dad cry once, and that was when they told him they were going to take my leg.

Janet Lanigan: From the very start, my parents gave me the choice whether to take chemotherapy or not. I don't know what would have happened if I had said no, but I always felt like it was my choice. They never pushed.

Dana Ensley: My mother tends to worry, so if I have a headache I try not to tell her. But it's best to just get it out in the open. Tell them. A lot of times when I had something wrong with me and I didn't tell, it got worse. Then I wished I had told them earlier so they could have gotten something done.

Millie Thomas: I think it would have been much, much more difficult for everybody if we'd hidden our feelings. If you're not honest about what you're feeling, you can't help anything. If you tell everybody you're okay and you're not, you can just kill yourself with emotions you kept inside.

Alice Demick: It's a guilty feeling to put your parents through that agony of seeing you sick. But it's just the way it is. I'd tell my mother how sorry I was, and she'd say, "No, no. We really love you, and we want you here no matter how much we have to go through. You're my kid, and I'm going to stay with you until the going's gone."

Columbus McRae: I often pretend I feel better than I do. That's what helps me carry on. I had a friend in the hospital who died, and then his mother had a heart attack and died. That's why I don't want my mother to know I'm hurting. I hold it in. I know when she's worried it makes me feel bad. I don't like my mother to worry.

Wayne Pelron: If anything happens, even if you get a headache, they'll sit you down and make sure everything is okay. Before, if you got a headache, they'd just give you a few aspirins and send you to bed. They're very protective. So act the way you did before. Don't over-complain.

What About Brothers and Sisters?

Robert Needham: My little sister was six when I got leukemia. She didn't know what it was all about, but she knew I was gone all the time and sick. I really had her scared. When I finally got out of the hospital, I tried to prove to her that I was going to be all right, that I was home and I was going to be there.

Cheryl Hall: There was a boy in the hospital at the same time I was, about seventeen, who got septicemia, a blood infection, and he just never really bounced back. He was really sick. But he had a little sister, too, my sister's age. And she and my sister got along so well because they knew how it was to have an older brother and sister who had cancer. They could talk to each other about how they felt when Mom or Dad had to go away or when the smaller one had to stay with a neighbor. They were just great for each other. And when he died, I think my sister was more shocked than I was. It was like my sister had lost a friend, too, because she wouldn't be seeing this little girl at the hospital anymore. And she was so upset. I didn't know what to say to her.

Tim Sperandio: My brother really got left out a lot. People always treated me special. I felt sorry for my brother, but I never said anything. It makes you feel guilty when you get more attention. And it made my brother mad at me for it. He used to say, "I'm gonna go around and tell everybody that you're bald." But when guys would come around and make cracks at me, he always stuck up for me. I was ashamed to have it happen, but I was too weak to do anything but watch.

Sometimes my brother got punished for something he didn't start. I'd go up to my room and take it out on myself.

At school I'd try to control my temper, and a good part of the time I did. But when you go through school for a whole day with kids making cracks at you, the first place you let it out is at home. I always tried to stick up for my own problems. I didn't like to come home and cry to my mom about which kids made fun of me. So I'd come home and gripe. It was hard on Joe, my brother. He's one of those kids with an outgoing personality, grins all the time. But he didn't know if he could talk to me or not. It was hard for everybody to cope with what I had.

Jeremy Varick: I'm the middle boy, and I was adopted. And one thing that makes me mad is that my little brother doesn't really understand. He thinks when my mom and I go off on these trips to the clinic, we're having fun. He's only eleven now, and he still doesn't realize that when we go down there it's not fun. When he gets mad, he always says my mom and dad don't care about him. They only stay around me all the time. But that's not true.

Jill Chapman: When my younger sister came to see me in the hospital, all she saw was the good stuff: the flowers, watching TV whenever I wanted, candy. While at home she was getting carted around to Grandma's and to the neighbor's, and *she* was washing all the dishes. She really got the bad end of the deal, and she was mad. She didn't like it at all.

But one day I told her what it was like to have a bone marrow. I told her the needles look like ice picks and that two doctors have to get on top and push it into your backbone. That was a shock, I think, for her. When she understood it wasn't all fun and games for me, she realized she wouldn't want it, either. It wasn't worth it.

Alice Demick: When your brothers and sisters tease you and call you the baby and say, "If it weren't for you . . . ," they don't realize that it makes you think, "Well, *really*, if it weren't for me . . ." It got to me.

Columbus McRae: Lots of times I think, "Why did it have to be me causing my mother all this trouble?" I can't help it because I got sick. Sometimes my brother and sisters throw that up in my face, that I'm making my mother suffer. I take long walks alone and talk it over with myself.

Sandy Brubaker: I don't think I really broke down about having my arm amputated until I had to tell my younger brother. He loves athletics like I do, so it was really hard for him to take. But the first thing I did when I got the bandages off was to try to learn to water ski again. I let him coach me about how to balance. It was something we could do together to show him that I was the same person he used to beat up. I wasn't fragile. And because I could accept it and go on, so could he.

School: Strange Looks, Stray Glances

Sheldon Masline: The biggest problem I've got now is being talked about. You know, people point you out all the time. You've just got to be able to cope with it.

Jill Chapman: I just wish people could take it in and know what it is to have cancer. That would be enough for me. But people sit around when I tell them things, and their eyes get real big and they go, "Oh, my gosh." It's like I'm telling them a gory story, like a freak story they can get their kicks on. It entertains *them,* but it doesn't help me.

Kenneth Lee Marsh: When I first went back to school, my friends would look at me like they were saying, "Are you the same?" But I told them if they had something they wanted to ask me, I'd tell them. Some of them told me later they thought I was just going to keel over. They thought there wasn't any cure for it. There's not a cure for it, but certain medicines work against it. If I can go three and a half years, I think I *will* be cured. And now my friends see I'm healthy, and they just figure there's nothing wrong with me. People I tell now think I'm kidding when I say I've got leukemia. I look just as healthy as anybody else.

Jeremy Varick: Some kids I'd tell would act stupid and say, "Eww," and move away, and say, "I don't want to catch it." But as you get older you know more and more about it, and so when kids ask you, "What's wrong? Why do you go to the doctor all the time?" you say, "Well, I have leukemia."

And usually they ask you right off, "Is it contagious?"

You just say, "No, it's not. It's a blood disease. It's in my blood."

I used to have to go to pathology every Thursday in the middle of math class. And the next day the kids would come up and ask, "Why'd you leave?"

And I'd say, "I had to go to the doctor." And I'd have to end up explaining it to them. But when it got toward the end of the year, I'd get up and everybody'd kind of wave "bye" because they all knew where I was going.

Sheldon Masline: When I first got it my friends kind of slacked up from hanging around me. And until I started reading about cancer, I thought I had caught it from my mom. So I told my friends, "You know, cancer is not a catchy thing, like chicken pox. Cancer is not like that." Now my friends know I have cancer, and they know I have Hodgkin's Disease. But they treat me like one of them, and that helps a whole bunch. They try to show me that I'm all right, and I try to show them that I am.

Brian McCalpin: I think teachers should understand that because I have leukemia I might not always feel so good. Just recently I've been feeling like maybe I could get away with saying, "Why should I?" But I try not to. I just want to act like the rest of the kids.

Jill Chapman: I tried out for a musical at school. I had been sick the year before, but I'd been off chemotherapy six months. I knew I could do it, and I knew there weren't a whole lot of other girls who could. My music teacher had always been really understanding about my being sick, but after the first try-outs, when they narrowed it down to the cut list, my name wasn't on the list. I was flabbergasted. So I asked the teacher, "What were the qualifications for that last cut list?"

He took me out into the hall, and he asked me how I was doing. And I said, "Fine. What do you mean?"

And he said, "Well, we can't . . . if you got sick."

I said, "How could you do that to me? There's nothing wrong with me. I don't limp; I don't do anything funny."

I was so upset with him. He was the one I thought understood. He understood too much. And the next day my name was on the list, and I made the part. There are always people I care about who care about me who are just misinformed, who just don't know how well I'm doing.

Cheryl Hall: I go through periods of insecurity at school because I feel like an outsider. I don't care about being part of the "in" crowd, but I like to have a circle of friends.

Anonymous: I had problems with people who couldn't understand. Nobody at school would ever come up to me and say, "Why did you lose your hair? Why are you always sick?" I just went home and sat down and cried about it. I never—which was a mistake—I never came out and said, "Well, I have a problem. Quit making fun of me." I put up with it and just let people run me around. But now I say my piece.

Brian McCalpin: I think sometimes that my classmates are scared that I'm going to die. I feel a little uneasy bringing it up. But if they ask, I feel pretty free to talk about it.

Frances Grimes: The school I'm going to this year has a funny rule that you can't wear scarves. They don't allow them. I agreed with them and said I'd wear a wig. The second day I was there, one of the girls asked me if I had a wig on. I said, "Yes, what's it to you?"

She said, "Uh, I just wanted to know."

I had to have a scarf on because the wig would slip off, my head was so slick. Then later she yanked it off my head. I kind of swung, and when I did I hit the teacher instead of her. I didn't hit her, because the teacher grabbed me. She saw the girl pull the wig off. She got suspended for two weeks. It made me mad, made me really want to hit her. I was angry inside; and I wanted it to come out, but it didn't. I'm glad it didn't because I would have said something I'd have regretted.

Robert Needham: When I went back to school, I looked a lot different. People in the hall didn't even recognize me. But that year I went out for football, and I made the team. That just goes to show you that you can come back through it. You can make it.

Wayne Pelron: I've done several talks for science class about leukemia and cancer in general. It really helps. It gives me a chance to let people know that I'm not a freak.

Alane Morehouse: When you go back to school, sometimes people think you've skipped. They can't believe you were that sick. They think you're on hard drugs because your eyes get all red. And when you go back there's always a lot of work to catch up on. I felt like I was *sick,* so why should I have to make up the work? But then I realized that if I didn't make it up I might fail, and then I'd have to do it all over again.

At first I wouldn't take my scarf off. I felt insecure without it. But now I feel out of place with it.

My friends helped. They pushed me to do stuff. I ride at a stable nearby, and my teacher there kept saying, "Come on, Alane, I know you can do it." That made me feel good. One thing I hate is to be pampered. I hate for people to say, "Poor Alane." I don't want my friends to say, "Are you all right? Can you do this?"

Tracy Klinko: Most people who don't know about cancer think that kids with cancer can't do anything other kids can do. They don't know that we're just the same, and we can do anything everybody else can do. You just have to get in there and do it, and tell them you can do it.

Valerie Nelcamp: One thing that really helped me, especially with my peers at school, was a sincere friendliness. I appreciated it when people treated me just like one of the gang. The kids who knew that I had had cancer and that I had lost my leg, but still accepted me for who I was and what I was, who looked to the inside and not so much to the outward appearances, were invaluable.

Anonymous: For seven months I had a tutor. When I got back to school, I vowed I'd make up for all the things I'd missed. I didn't even know about homecoming week. I didn't have any idea there were so many basketball games in high school.

Tracy Klinko: I lost some school, but I took a placement test so I could go on. Sometimes when you go back, the kids can't believe you were really sick. I was in the third, fourth, and fifth grades when this happened to me, and when my parents came in and talked to the teacher, it made me feel little. Like you can't handle it yourself. I'd rather handle it myself.

Tim Sperandio: I had a tutor who would come in, and all she was interested in was talking. She didn't care about me or my school work. She tried to make me cheat. She came in and looked at my math and saw I was having trouble with it, so she got out the answer book and opened it and said, "Copy this."

I'm surprised I passed the seventh grade. I felt, "Oh gosh, I'm gonna flunk this grade." I fell behind. Some of the work I couldn't do without her help. But I made A's and B's, and I was surprised. I think they should have given me what I deserved, and I didn't deserve anything over a D.

When I went back to school I had lost all my hair, and we had just moved from Colorado to Missouri. I got a lot of cracks. Two girls would be walking down the hall, and they'd start talking together, laughing at me, and turn around and point and stuff. It made me mad. I'd come home a lot of times feeling really mad over it. I didn't like it, but I'd try to explain it to some of them. The ones who were interested didn't make fun of me, and dealt with it, but the others just laughed. I guess they were ignorant. They didn't like me because I was different. Kids are pretty silly about things like that.

When I looked so bad, and people would ask, I'd tell them I have leukemia. And they'd go, "How long do you have to live?" It was always that. One day a kid sitting in study hall with me goes, "How long are you gonna live?"

So I had to go through the whole thing, tell him how I got it, and the medicines I had to take, and he goes, "You gonna live?"

And I said, "As far as I know I am."

Now this year they're saying, "Look at all the hair you've got! You look a lot healthier." A few teachers couldn't get over the fact that I looked so good. I mean they really commented about me.

Cheryl Hall: I don't know if everybody has this problem, but at school kids smoke in the bathroom. So you're walking down the hall, and you can see the cigarette smoke coming out of the bathroom. One day I walked in there and made a fool of myself, but I was so mad. These kids—the same ones who signed the cards sent to me in the hospital—were in there smoking. These were people who had said to me, "My gosh, how did you do it? You fought and overcame cancer. It's a miracle you're alive." And they're standing around *smoking*. I said to them, "If you guys don't put out those cigarettes, I swear I'm going to take every one of you and put your heads through the cement wall. How can you be so stupid, after you've seen all I've been through? How can you come in here and smoke?"

Dating

Valerie Nelcamp: Because I have had cancer, I think that people are afraid to develop a close relationship with me. I know some of the kids say, "Well, don't get real close to her because something could happen, and we'd end up hurt."

I have another problem because of my leg. I worry about whether a boy will accept me as I am. I know society places a great deal of importance on physical beauty. But when they amputated my leg, they didn't take my personality. I am still a person, and I think I still have a lot to give. Even so, some people might not be able to look beyond that physical handicap.

Sandy Brubaker: When I was in the hospital, there was a guy three years older than I am, a good friend who had known me a while. And he came to the hospital a couple of days after my arm was amputated, but he wouldn't come upstairs. He told me later, "Sandy, I wanted to come see you. There was so much I wanted to say to you. But I got in that car and just cried. I couldn't face you. I couldn't face the fact that you've got it. It's so close. It's home. It's around *me*. There a possibility. . . ."

I think that's what's happening when guys don't come see you in the hospital.

Eddy Kimball: I had this girl I really liked, and I was taking chemotherapy at the time and was out of it on Friday nights. I had a lot of homework. I was taking some pretty tough classes and just couldn't take her out during the week. She hung by me, and now that I am not getting that chemotherapy in the summer, we talk to each other almost every night. I just want to say, if they hang by you, they really understand.

Anonymous: With friends, it doesn't make any difference with or without a leg. Guys are going to like you anyway, if they're your friend. In fact, they'll like you more. If you go on and live life without worrying about it, they'll see you have courage and they'll admire you. They don't look at that (cancer). They look at your personality. They don't care about the other. If they do, they'll avoid you altogether. If they're taking you out because they feel sorry for you, you'll know by the way they act. Usually, though, the guys I've gone out with took me because they liked me as a person.

Anonymous: One girl at school would tell every guy who showed any interest in me that I had cancer. She'd say, "You better not run very fast or you'll come down with your cancer again," and things like that.

Most guys don't really know what cancer is, and they take off. But some guys are really understanding. They don't care about your scars.

Kenneth Lee Marsh: I tell myself, "There's more than one fish in the ocean." There's more than one girl I can go out with. If they don't want to got out with me because I have leukemia, that's all right with me. Some girls I don't even tell. Then other girls already know about it. Some get turned off by it. They think, "Well, he's got a disease."

I just don't let it bother me.

Alice Demick: I think it's unnecessary to tell a guy about your cancer when you first know him. But before it gets too serious, I think they should know how your life's been. If they love you, they won't reject you because of it.

Anonymous: If I felt serious about a guy, I'd tell him that I have cancer but that it's not contagious, that I'm not weird. It's just a malfunction in your cells. They didn't come out exactly perfect.

Lisa Robison: I used to date only certain guys. I wouldn't date guys with bad reputations. But you'd be surprised how nice those guys can be. All my friends, other girls, are missing out on these great guys they think are so tacky. Now (after the relapse), if anybody asks me out, I'll go, because I think now if I don't get out and go I might miss something.

I take a lot more interest in people's lives, and I remember things more clearly. Little things. I pay more attention to what's going on.

People treat you a whole lot different if you tell them you have cancer, though. One guy I met this summer just disappeared. I never saw him again after I told him.

Anonymous: I have one guy I think about all the time. I'm ashamed to say this, but I thought to myself when I got sick, "Well, now that they almost lost me, maybe he'll appreciate me more." He *did* pay more attention to me, but he still treated me like a friend. He never called me or anything. He didn't even write a card.

Anonymous: We couldn't talk about it. My boy friend wasn't ready for it. We talked about marriage and he said he loved me, but he just didn't know if he could marry me.

And I said, "Good grief, why not? I don't understand this. You love me with all this other stuff (chemotherapy), why can't you marry me?"

He said, "Well, I would just hate to lose you."

I said, "Well, I could lose you, too. We both take a big chance. You can't talk about odds because everybody dies, period."

But what I was thinking was, "You coward!"

He could accept the fact that I'd been sick and that it had enriched my life, but he couldn't believe that my life would last. He was not allowing me to talk about it. And that intimidated me. I knew I wasn't going to change his mind. He didn't have any faith in me.

What If I'm Sterile?

Anonymous: I had radiation to my left pelvic area, so I had to sign papers because my ovary would be involved, and they said it probably wouldn't function. I know it doesn't now. For a long time my periods weren't straight, but now they are. They're even regular, now. I never thought that would happen. It took a couple of years. So it would seem like I could [have children], but I don't want to. I think I'd feel terribly guilty if I had a child and there was something wrong with it, for any reason. I'd feel terribly guilty. I don't want to do that. I don't feel I have the right to do that. If children become important, I think I will be satisfied with adoption.

I know the fear I would have, carrying that baby. I don't want that fear. I can never understand why it's so important to other girls to have a family. My thing is getting through college. I want to graduate from college, then get a job. I want to help other kids like me, to get to know them and talk to them [about cancer].

Debra Vehlewald: They tell me if I stay on the chemotherapy I'll be all right, as long as I'm on it. But I want to get off of it. All I'm thinking about now is whether I'm going to live long enough to have a family. Have a family, raise my kids, just like everybody else. It's really upsetting that you don't know if you can or not. It makes you stop and think. My girl friend has a two-year-old, and I sit and play with her and just think, "I just hope I can have one like her." It's affected me a great deal.

I want to know what's going to happen. You just don't know. I want to know, and I want to know now. But you just don't. You can't find out.

Anonymous: When the doctor told me I might not be able to have kids, I cried and cried. I've always wanted to have kids. That was my one dream of my life.

Sheldon Masline: I've thought, "Will I ever be able to have children?" I want to have one or two kids. If I can't have one, I'll probably adopt one. I'd be glad to do that. No matter what, I want to have me a little son or daughter running around.

Millie Thomas: One of the things that helped me the most was the fact of test tube babies. I don't know what possibilities it has for chemotherapy patients, but I think it gives girls a lot of hope.

Tim Sperandio: All my life I feel I've been used as a medical guinea pig. The doctors never told me the consequences (of cancer drugs). After I started reading about them, I knew what was keeping me from growing and keeping my hair from growing. They also sterilized me. Now I'll never be able to have children. To have someone take away your power to have children, it upset me a lot. It really makes me mad. But there's nothing that can be done now. That's all ruined for me.

Cheryl Hall: Some girls worry about getting pregnant, but I'm really scared I won't be able to have kids. I'm afraid that when I meet the right guy, he's going to reject me because of that. That's got to be the biggest worry I have right now. My doctor told me that they don't know what chemotherapy does. It doesn't do the same thing to everybody. He said it might be a long time before you have your period, it might come back right now, it might not ever come back. And he warned me of the danger of getting pregnant while you're on chemotherapy. He said it's just like taking LSD.

Alane Morehouse: I don't worry about not having children. I figure I'll be through with my chemotherapy and will be able to have kids. My doctor never told me anything about that, and I just never did worry about it.

Alice Demick: I'm not sure how I feel about having kids. I don't know if they could get what I had. I don't know if I could handle having sick kids.

If my kids had what I had, it would bring back a lot of memories that would touch close. I would know exactly what they were going through. I think I would tend to feel sorry instead of understanding. And understanding's what you need.

Martha Billings: I want to go ahead and have children. When you get pregnant, that's a lot of hormones changing, and a lot of things are changing. I've thought about that. (I never received any drug treatments after my mastectomy.) It could be dangerous. But it might not. I could have picked up the cancer from some chemical, something like that. My gynecologist has never expressed any fear about it. It makes sense, though—I mean, it's such a time of change for your body—it could happen. But I think I'd have to have some kind of cancer starting before . . . I'm just going ahead and take my chances.

Attitude—Keep Your Chin Up!

Jill Chapman: I have to use self-discipline as much as I can make myself. Self-discipline is a must. The only time I can afford to get depressed is when I'm feeling really good and know that I could not feel good like this again. I could be sick again. That's when I get depressed—usually when everything is going well. When things get bad, to me it's something to get over, it's not something to worry about. I can't just let go. Because if I let go, first I'd waste time, and second, I'd make dumb mistakes.

Anonymous: When you are depressed about some little thing, any little problem, then one thought leads to another and you start thinking about your cancer. You've got to fight that.

Anonymous: The first thing your friends want to do is pamper you. You've got to say, "No." You can't let them do that because the more you let them pamper you, the more spoiled you get and the less you want to do for yourself. You've got to tell them, "No, I'm still a person, and I can still do everything I did before, and if I need help, I'll ask for it." And if you just tell them like that, then it's fine.

Another thing: You have to get ahold of your friends after you get out of the hospital, because they'll be afraid to bother you. They're afraid they're going to upset you or hurt your feelings.

If you keep a positive attitude, it inspires people around

you, too. After the newspaper ran a story about my losing my leg, people on the street would come up and say, "I've seen you in the paper, and I think you're doing a great job." That makes you feel good.

Tracy Klinko: I never used to pray, talk to Him, stuff like that. But when you go through cancer you change a lot. Your attitude changes. It's like you're a whole new person. After you've been through it, you're a lot more grown up. After I got out of the hospital I had the urge to go on and do the things I wanted to do before; it made me realize that I might not have the chance to do them later. So every day it urges me on to do the things I want to do.

Dana Ensley: Positive attitude is very important. If you think to yourself, "I'm gonna get better," and "I'm not gonna let this thing get me down," then it won't.

New Perspectives

Sandy Brubaker: When they told me I would lose my arm, I made a promise to myself. From that point on, I knew I had to make more of my life. If you know you can do something yourself, then do it. If you think you can't, try to *find* a way.

Kenneth Lee Marsh: It gives you more to think about, more to respect yourself for. People who are healthy will never know what it is to go through something like this.

Columbus McRae: I think cancer changed my whole personality. I used to be mean, but now I'm more sensitive to things people say.

Valerie Nelcamp: I have come to appreciate life, and I see more good in life than I ever used to. I believe we should live one day at a time but plan like we are going to be here forever.

Robert Needham: You can look at it this way: You might have cancer, but think of it as an adventure. You can learn a lot. If you ask the doctors, they'll show you how to do the bone marrows and blood tests. When you find out you have cancer, you either grow up right there or become a baby for the rest of your life. Like they say, you've got to grin and bear it. Living becomes a gift, too. Life becomes something precious. There's a lot of comfort in knowing what could have happened to me that didn't.

Dana Ensley: I know I'm a stronger person because of cancer, and I know my parents are stronger. Especially my mom. She can see how it is for kids who are sick. Before I got sick, we only saw one world, and that was a world where everybody was all right. If anybody was sick, it was a cold or a virus. But now we see this other world, these kids going through things they have to go through. In realizing that there is this other world, we've all gotten stronger and closer to the Lord.

Millie Thomas: The possibilities of losing my hair and becoming sterile and dying never hit me until I read those sheets that tell you all the side effects of the drugs. And then it just washed over me like a wave. I couldn't look my doctor in the face. But in about fifteen minutes it was all over. I think I was feeling sorry for myself at that time. But there were so many other people worse off than I was, even in the next room, that if I did catch myself feeling sorry for myself, I'd just think of all the things it *could* have been instead of Hodgkin's.

Columbus McRae: It helps to talk with other people who have had cancer. I have gone in and talked to patients at the hospital. This one boy wanted to kill himself. I told him there wasn't any need for that. I asked him if he loved his family and he said, "Yes."

I said, "By killing yourself you're not going to help them. You're only making yourself worthless to them. They are the ones that will have to take it then."

It stopped him. And it made me feel that I can kind of talk people out of things. It made me feel like I could do some good. Since I've been through it, I feel I can help other people get through it.

Faith

Alice Demick: Life has many crosses, and you just have to pick them up and carry them. But God's not going to give you a bigger cross than you can handle.

Anonymous: Sure, I said, "Why *me*?" But I decided God had something planned for me, or He wouldn't have let me live at all.

Robert Needham: I'm a Christian, so I feel that the Lord is going to use this in some way that I can tell somebody else, "Hey, look, I was going to die and the Lord pulled me through, and He can pull you through. He can pull you out."

Anonymous: Have you ever tried to wish it on somebody else? I try to stop myself and think, "No, don't ever wish that on anybody, no matter how terrible they are." But I know if they got it they'd go crazy, they wouldn't know how to handle it. I think if you get it, God had a reason for giving it to you. Maybe He did this to me so I could help other kids. I think He gives it to people like a test of faith. And He wouldn't give it to anybody He thought couldn't handle it.

Dana Ensley: The most important thing to me is that I have been able to see myself as a different person. I've grown closer to the Lord. I used to put some things, other things, before Him. I wasn't as dedicated. Now, I get my positive attitude from God, and from what the Bible says: Put all thy trust in

Thee. That's what I believe. You may not be able to see God, but I know He's there.

You've got a lot better chance if you've got that fight within you. But if you carry around negative thoughts and say, "What's the use? I give up," it's just gonna take longer and you may not get better. That's the way I look at it. Some people find it just within themselves, but I find it from God.

TOO CLOSE FOR COMFORT: STRAIGHT TALK ABOUT DYING

The Relapse: Here We Go Again

Lisa Robison: When my friends sit around talking about what they'll be doing ten years from now, I know. Lisa's not going to be here. That's the way I think. It just seems so crazy. I'll be dead by that time.

I *would* like to stick around and see what everybody's doing. You know you're not going to be here and if you fool yourself into thinking you are, you're stupid. It's just stupid. It all depends on the prognosis—how bad you are in the first place. You can have two or three relapses. That's not the thing.

If your first relapse comes after two or three years, you'll live a whole lot longer. But I was only in remission five months. That's what gets me. Besides the actual part about being in your casket and all your friends standing around crying, I don't want to leave. I've got too many things going for me. My life is just getting started.

Anybody who has a terminal illness will tell you that dying is something that goes through your mind a hundred times a day. You're always thinking that maybe they'll do something about it. Maybe they won't. It makes you more aware of things like the Jerry Lewis Telethon to help people out who are pretty much in the same boat. You feel more charitable toward people.

It makes you realize that you haven't got much time left and what you do now they're going to remember you by. That helps out. You want to make each day nice. The way I see it, you just live for today.

Jeremy Varick: When you get a relapse you say to yourself, "Oh no, here it comes." I've had three relapses. All you can do is hope to go as long as you can without having a relapse. But when you get a relapse it's bad news. It is. And you usually cry a little and then start thinking stupid, like "Why me?" Then you get over it. You've got to realize it's started again. My mom keeps telling me, "We can conquer this." I do a lot more thinking than I used to. You're always thinking, "What's going to happen?"

Anonymous: We spent all that money, and then it came back. I felt like asking for a refund.

Sheldon Masline: All I can think about is that it will keep coming back, no matter what. If you get it once, you know what it's going to be like the second time around. I discovered my first relapse myself. When the lymph nodes in my neck started swelling, I could feel them and I got scared. Four days later they said it had come back. I thought to myself, "They didn't do a very good job. If they aren't going to do a good job, they shouldn't do it at all. All the medicine was for nothing. It came back."

It's terrifying. I think about how it could just start spreading faster and faster and just take me like that. The best part about having it is that you have a half-and-half chance of living. You can be treated, and hopefully, it could go away. I can't just give up, though. I haven't seen everything I want to see, and I thought this cancer was going to keep me from doing things. But it hasn't. Everywhere I go, I want to keep a smile on everybody's face for me. I want them to know me. I wouldn't want to die and have them say, "Who was he?" At night I lay there thinking about where I'm going to go when I die. I'm like some kind of walking time bomb. I make my peace with Him everyday.

Jill Chapman: I think about a relapse a lot. In fact, the older I get the more I think about it. It's so unfair, to be healthy and to have to get sick again. I like to think I can side-step it and go on, yet I realize the possibilities of getting sick again, and I want to be ready for it. Each time you have a relapse, you approach it from a different angle. It's not like starting all over again. I think fear is really not knowing. It is for me. When I don't know if it's coming back, I'm scared. I know the possibilities. If I get sick again, it could be an organ. Suppose it were my spinal cord, my vertebrae? If I couldn't think, I'd just as soon die.

Frances Grimes: Whenever I get an ache or a pain, I just sit on my bed and pray that it's not that. Anything but that. I wonder if it's going to start all over again.

Sandy Brubaker: A recurrence, just knowing it could come back anytime, is like carrying a five hundred-pound weight around with you.

Dana Ensley: When I had my first relapse, I had thought I was doing so well. It was like my world had just crashed down around me. I know I told a friend of mine, "I don't think I have got enough fight left in me anymore." That's scary.

But after I had time to think more, it just seemed like the fight within me was greater than it had been before. It made me want to fight even harder. Don't ever give up. Keep fighting. It may look bad and you may think, "Well, what's the use?" but really, it's worth it. I love my family and my friends, and I'm just not ready to leave them. Believing in God can really help. I don't think about dying. There's no use to now. What I'm thinking is to keep on fighting, keep on living. I figure I'm going to be around for a long time. I'll believe that until I draw the last breath. I'll always believe it.

Alane Morehouse: When I had the first relapse I just couldn't believe that it had spread. It spread to my head—to my brain. I was having real bad headaches from the pressure of the cancer spreading. I was frustrated. I said, "Why me?" I felt I didn't do anything to deserve this. But if I have to live with it, there's nothing I can do about it. Just make the best of it. I think about running away a lot, but I'm scared that if I miss a lot of medicine I'm going to get sick again. And if I was to die, how would my friends and family feel? What would they think? They'd think I was a weakling or something.

Brian McCalpin: You know, when you're well you don't really think about having the disease at all. When you feel good it's easy to forget about it.

When I first got leukemia I didn't know that much about it. I was ten. I just thought, "This is the way God wants it to be." I had treatments for three years, and I was in remission for two before I had a relapse. But this time I was a lot more scared. I knew what the treatments would be like. I know a lot more about the disease and what it can do. And I've thought, "What if I don't get better?" Younger kids, in a naive sense, have a much easier time believing they'll get well permanently. I know when I was so sick the first time I kept thinking, "With God I can get better." But then I'd think, "If God wants me to get better, why am I so sick?"

Anonymous: When I had my first operation, they didn't say it could come back. I thought it was all gone. But apparently it wasn't. I only had a month to go, and I would be finished with chemotherapy when I found out I had a recurrence. I got really down—deep down depressed—because without asking, I knew I would have to start chemotherapy over again. It meant I'd have to go through another operation not knowing how it was going to turn out.

Then I had a second recurrence. It really hurt. That meant another amputation. But since I have had it twice before, I feel if it happens to me again I'll be ready for it.

Heaven knows if it is going to come back or not, but if it does, it might come back where they can't do anything for you. They've told me that it could happen anytime. It could happen to anyone. So I'm ready for a recurrence. I don't know if I'm ready for taking chemotherapy again. That's a decision I'll make when I have to.

Karen Jepsen: I would hope and pray that anyone who has to face a relapse would have the right attitude and would be willing to start chemotherapy or radiation one more time. It takes friends, family, and a faith that enables you to want to go on living enough to fight. At first I questioned whether I was up to induction and the possibility of radiation and losing my hair again. But I was shown so much love and support that by the time induction had started I was more than ready to fight it one more time, and it's going great.

Alternatives to Treatment

Linda Von Seggers: When I first got sick, so many people told me to go to Russia, go to Mexico, take Laetrile. My mother was going insane because people were calling up and telling her, "You should be going to St. Judes or Houston or here or there." My mother asked *me*. She said, "Now, if you want to do this, it's up to you." And we got all the information on Laetrile—that was one big thing—and looked over it, and I said, "Mom, I'm doing so well right now on chemotherapy I can see results. I've never seen any people cured with Laetrile, or even doing super good. So I want to stick with what I'm doing." I think I would be really scared to go off treatment. But I had a lot of people telling me about beet juice diets and water diets and all these.

Tim Sperandio: I did a lot of reading over the summer. A friend has a big library, and I just picked up these books: *How to Prevent and Gain Remission from Cancer* and *World Without Cancer, The Story of Vitamin B-17* [G. Edward Griffin, American Media, Westlake Valley, Calif.]. They convinced me that the medicine is just poison. It was keeping me from growing, and I was always getting sick. I decided that fresh fruits and vegetables—and not chemicals—can cure me of leukemia. When they put that medicine into your veins, it stays there forever. It made me act like a monster. On chemotherapy I felt like Dr. Jekyll and Mr. Hyde. So I called the doctors and told them I didn't want the drugs anymore. I told them that I'm just eating fruits and vegetables. The doctors said it would come back within three weeks to a month, maybe a little longer. It's been eighteen months and nothing's come back, and I'm still doing what I want to do. In my opinion I'm doing good. I'm healthy. I feel a lot healthier than I did, even before I had leukemia.

Finding Peace

Columbus McRae: I thought I might die many times. When I first had leukemia they called all my family from upstate and everywhere else to come. The doctors told me that I might not ever go home. But I said, "As long as the good Lord's upstairs, I'm not going nowhere." I knew God would help me if I asked Him to, and so I did. I prayed and pulled on up. As long as I know the good Lord, I can go on.

Sandy Brubaker: People say, "What are you going to do when you grow up?" I sometimes wonder what I'll do if I don't.

Alice Demick: I knew I was going to die, I just didn't know when. But I knew it was getting closer and closer. I was really dissatisfied with myself in that I would get upset at people who asked me how I was feeling. It was plain to see that I felt rotten. It bothered me that I was disrespectful to my mother when I'm not that way with anybody else. I was not ready to die because of that. I'd pinpointed it to that. Otherwise I didn't see anything wrong with my life or why I should go to hell. That was the only thing. Then Sister Margaret convinced me that everybody makes mistakes and that Jesus would forgive me that mistake. Everybody dies sometime. You're not condemned just because you're sick.

Cheryl Hall: It aggravates me when people say cancer is terminal. After all, *life* is terminal.

Sherry Parton: I worry about dying. It's stupid because I figure I'll *know* when I'm going to die. I'll just have a feeling, and what has to be will be. I can't stop my life from going on. If you can just get your mind off of it. There's no use worrying. It can only upset you more. Take one day at a time, and do your best. That's all you've got to do. That's all you *can* do.

Tracy Klinko: I was dead for ten minutes. Cardiac arrest. I had kidney failure, and I was on dialysis and a bowel bypass because I had a bunch of tumors and they had to cut them out. When you die it's like being blocked off in a room with no one to talk to. Nothing to hear. Nothing to see. Just black and quiet. It's like floating in nothingness. It's like you're asleep, but no dreams. I even got some cards that said stuff like, "Sorry to see you go." But I didn't pay much attention to them. In the movies it seems like the people always die. But it's not like that. Most people who have cancer don't die. They should have one about a kid who lives. Then kids who have just gotten cancer will think, "If that kid can live and be on TV maybe I can live."

Lisa Robison: There's a big difference in knowing and believing [you may die]. My sister knew it and Tom, my boy friend. They love me, and what they see is that I was a cheerleader, I played basketball, touch football, and now I'm laying up in the hospital with an IV in my arm. It really tears them up. They just can't understand why I'm up there just about dead. I had the biggest problem with my best friend. She could not realize that I was very sick and that I was on the verge of death. She couldn't handle it, and so she wouldn't come, she wouldn't see me. I made a special effort to go see her. And I said to her, "Look me in the face." And she did, and her eyes were full of tears. And I said, "Look, I may live for years." After that she realized that just because you've got it doesn't mean you're going to die.

Bowing Out: The Funeral/How to Die

Jill Chapman: Some people do well at dying, and some people don't do so good. A little girl who just died was excellent at it. She planned her funeral. She had things she wanted done. She loved Elvis Presley, so there had to be an Elvis Presley song. She picked it out. She responded to other people's love. People loved her a lot and let her know, and she responded to that. Sometimes if you let yourself withdraw, it makes it harder on the people around you. If I were dying, I know I would want to push people away and say, "Don't watch me like this, don't watch me dying." But she didn't. Her family didn't feel that she had rejected them afterwards. They felt she needed to have them there.

Anonymous: My biggest goal is that when I know I'm going to die I want to be able to accept it. I don't want to die hard, but if I have to die painfully I want to be able to accept it. The more painful it is, the harder it's going to be to accept. I know I'll fight as long as I can, but when I know the time has come, there's nothing more I can do, I want everyone to know it's okay. I'm worried most about my mother.

Robert Needham: At one point they gave me so many hours to live. I just told myself I was going home. I was bound and determined to go home, and something inside me kept on saying, "You're gonna go home; you're gonna go home." I think if I had said, "I can't hold on any longer," I would have gone ahead and died.

Columbus McRae: Once I gave up hope, and even told them I was going to die. Looked like something in my head was saying, "Yeah, you want to die." Then things changed. I hit myself in the head. It sounds dumb, but I did it. I picked up something and hit myself, to knock it out of my head.

Glossary, Further Readings, and Where To Go For Help

Glossary

Adjuvant chemotherapy—using chemotherapy in addition to surgery and/or radiation to treat cancer that may be spreading.

Antibiotic—a drug that can destroy disease germs or stop them from growing.

Antidote—a rescue drug given to counteract treatments to kill cancer cells.

Benign tumor—a nonmalignant tumor that is considered relatively harmless.

Biopsy—a minor operation in which a sliver of tissue is removed from a suspicious lump so that it can be examined under a microscope.

Bone marrow—the sponge-like tissue inside bones where blood cells are produced.

Bone marrow biopsy and aspiration—with a needle, the doctor withdraws a sample of bone marrow inside a patient's bone. The sample can then be studied at the laboratory to make sure it contains plenty of healthy cells.

Carcinogen—something that can cause cancer.

Carcinoma—a malignant cancer that begins in the covering tissues such as those found in the lining of the lungs and digestive tract.

CAT (Computerized Axial Tomography) Scan—a modern X-ray technique that gives pictures of the body in minute detail.

Chemotherapy—the treatment of cancer with drugs.

Chronic—long, drawn out; not acute.

Chronic myelogenous leukemia—a form of leukemia in which the leukemia cells come from the bone marow. An individual may live from one to twenty-five years or more with the disease.

Cobalt treatment—a common use of radiation as therapy for cancer confined to one area.

Combination chemotherapy—using two or more drugs together to treat cancer.

Comparative clinical trial—a planned experiment to determine the best treatment to use in future patients.

Cryosurgery—a super-cold surgery using nitrogen liquid injected with a probe.

Cured—a word used cautiously to describe cancer patients who have lived two to five years or more after treatment without evidence of active or recurrent disease.

Cytoplasm—all of the cell's plasma other than the nucleus.

Cytoxic—destructive to cells.

Granulocytes—white cells that fight infection by engulfing bacteria.

Hematologist—a doctor who specializes in the treatment of diseases of the blood.

Hemoglobin—the oxygen-carrying protein in red blood cells.

Hemangioma—a tumor composed of blood vessels.

Hodgkin's disease—cancer of the lymph system.

Immunotherapy—using the body's own defenses to fight cancer.

Laser—sharply focused beams of hot light.

Leukemia—cancer of the blood. With leukemia, the body has made too many white blood cells, which may be deformed and unable to fight infection. These crowd out the red blood cells and normal bone marrow production.

Leukemia virus—a virus found in animals, but not in humans, capable of causing leukemia.

Leukocytes—white blood cells.

Lymphocytes—cells formed in the lymph glands, the spleen and tonsils. Lymphocytes are a kind of white blood cell. They normally number from twenty-five to thirty percent of the total white cells. They may increase to ninety percent in lymphatic leukemia.

Lymphoid organs—these organs make up the body's defense system. They include the spleen (in the abdomen), the lymph nodes (in the neck, armpits, and groin), and the thymus (near the throat). They produce antibodies that work to repel foreign substances.

Lymphosarcoma—a cancer of the lymphatic system.

Macrophages—white blood cells that attack invading germs.

Malignant tumor—a tumor that keeps on growing. Cells from a malignant tumor can dislodge and be carried by the bloodstream to other parts of the body and become new tumors.

Melanoma—a malignant skin cancer.

Metastasis—the spread of cancer cells. A tumor is said to metastasize when a piece of it breaks away and rides in the bloodstream to another part of the body, where it may form a new tumor.

Mitotic inhibitors—drugs produced from the periwinkle plant, among them vincristine.

Mutation—a change in a gene, usually caused by radiation or chemicals.

Neuroblastoma—cancer of the nerves.

Neuroma—a tumor growing on a nerve, and in many cases, producing pain.

Oncologist—a doctor who specializes in the treatment of cancer.

Osteoma—a tumor composed of bone.

Osteogenic sarcoma—bone cancer.

Platelets—the part of the blood responsible for clotting.

Prognosis—a prediction the doctor makes about how a patient will do, based on the outcome of treatment on similar cases.

Protocol—a formal treatment plan.

Prosthesis—an artificial limb.

Radiation—a beam that can pass through objects that visible light cannot penetrate. From X rays come pictures of bones and organs beneath the skin.

Relapse—the return of a disease.

Remission—a marked improvement, or complete disappearance, of the cancer.

Retinoblastoma—a highly malignant tumor in the retina of the eye that usually runs in families. It occurs most often in young children.

Sarcoma—cancer in such connective tissues as bone, cartilage, and muscles.

Sedative—a drug given to sooth over-excited nerves.

Spinal tap—inserting a needle into the canal between the vertebrae (back bones) to withdraw fluid or inject medicine.

Tumor—a swelling or abnormal growth of tissues in the body. Some tumors are benign. They limit themselves to a certain region and do not spread elsewhere. Once removed, they do not grow again. Malignant tumors that are not completely removed can spread throughout the body, often destroying other tissues.

Further Reading

Books About People With Cancer

Alsop, Stewart. *Stay of Execution.* Philadelphia: Lippincott Co., 1973. Autobiographic account of battle with cancer.

Fox, Ray Errol. *Angela Ambrosia.* New York: Alfred A. Knopf, 1979. Story of teenaged girl's struggle with leukemia, over-protective parents, and impersonal hospital staff.

Gunther, John. *Death Be Not Proud.* New York: Harper & Row, 1971. A father's story of his son, who died of a brain tumor.

Ipswitch, Elaine. *Scot Was Here.* New York: Delacorte Press, 1979. Diary of a teenaged boy with Hodgkin's disease.

Klein, Norma. *Sunshine.* New York: Avon Publishers, 1974. Determined to leave something of herself behind for her daughter Jennifer, Lyn Helton, twenty, wrote this frank diary during the last months of her life. Her story was also told in the June 1972 *Reader's Digest.*

Lee, Laurel. *Walking Through the Fire:* A Hospital Journal. New York: Bantam, 1978. Brief, easy-to-read account of a young, pregnant woman's decision to postpone treatment for Hodgkin's disease until after the birth of her child. Positive, hopeful tone.

Lund, Doris. *Eric.* New York: Dell Books, 1976. At seventeen, Eric accepted his grim diagnosis with leukemia, yet went on to college, played soccer, took a cross-country trip, and fell in love before finally succumbing to the disease at twenty-two. A moving acount as told by his mother.

Books That Explain Cancer

There Is a Rainbow Behind Every Dark Cloud. Center for Attitudinal

Healing, Tiburon, California. Upbeat, direct book for kids dealing with life-threatening illnesses.

Baker, Lyn S. *You and Leukemia: A Day at a Time.* Rochester, Minn.: Mayo Comprehensive Cancer Center, 1976. Handbook on childhood leukemia, addressed to children nine and up. Clear, candid, supportive, and informative. Available from some clinics, or through the publisher, W. B. Saunders Company, West Washington Square, Philadelphia, Pennsylvania 19105

For a list of other books and pamphlets about cancer, write for *Readings on Cancer,* an annotated bibliography, free from the Office of Cancer Communications, National Cancer Institute, Bethesda, Maryland 20014.

Where to Go for Help

The Cancer Information Service answers questions about cancer, medical facilities in your area, possible sources of financial aid, and physician consultation services. Call toll-free 800-638-6694.

The American Cancer Society supports cancer research and treatment and supplies a wide range of literature to patients and their families.

Leukemia Society of America, Inc., a voluntary organization devoted to research funding, offers literature and financial assistance for drugs, blood, transportation, and X-ray treatment to out-patients with leukemia, the lymphomas, and Hodgkin's disease. Write National Headquarters, 211 East 43rd Street, New York, New York 10017 or call a local Leukemia Society agency.

The Cancer Information Clearinghouse keeps a running bibliography of films, audiovisuals, and publications categorized by subject. Write 7910 Woodmont Ave., Suite 1320, Bethesda, Maryland 20014. To hurry things along, ask specifically for information about childhood cancers and sources of financial assistance.

Candlelighters, Inc., a nationwide organization formed by parents of young cancer victims, publishes a newsletter and an annual cumulative bibliography of references of interest to members. To receive the newsletter, write Candlelighters, 123 C Street, S.E., Washington, D.C. 20003. Guidance and advice through this telephone number: 202-483-9100.

Ronald McDonald Houses provide an alternative to hospital chairs and expensive accommodations for families of seriously ill children.

Usually located near the hospital, a dozen of these homes have already opened. Others are planned. They offer a cheery atmosphere, understanding housemates, and kitchen facilities. Charge? Around five dollars a night. For more information write to A.D. Bud Jones, National Coordinator, Children's Oncology Services, Inc., 500 N. Michigan Ave., Chicago, Illinois 60611.

The Christian Bible Society is a nonprofit organization committed to the belief that all persons can benefit from reading the Bible. If you want a free Bible, write to the Christian Bible Society, Nashville, Tennessee 37210. They can also put you in touch with someone in your area who is willing to discuss spiritual matters with you.